TUBERCULOSIS THEN AND NOW

MCGILL-QUEEN'S/ASSOCIATED MEDICAL SERVICES STUDIES IN
THE HISTORY OF MEDICINE, HEALTH, AND SOCIETY

SERIES EDITORS: S.O. FREEDMAN AND J.T.H. CONNOR

Volumes in this series have financial support from Associated Medical
Services, Inc. (AMS). Associated Medical Services Inc. was established in
1936 by Dr Jason Hannah as a pioneer prepaid not-for-profit health-care
organization in Ontario. With the advent of medicare, AMS became a
charitable organization supporting innovations in academic medicine and
health services, specifically the history of medicine and health care, as
well as innovations in health professional education and bioethics.

Tuberculosis Then and Now

Perspectives on the History of an Infectious Disease

Edited by

FLURIN CONDRAU

and

MICHAEL WORBOYS

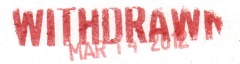
McGill-Queen's University Press
Montreal & Kingston • London • Ithaca

© McGill-Queen's University Press 2010

ISBN 978-0-7735-3600-5 (cloth)
ISBN 978-0-7735-3601-2 (paper)

Legal deposit first quarter 2010
Bibliothèque nationale du Québec

Printed in Canada on acid-free paper that is 100% ancient forest
free (100% post-consumer recycled), processed chlorine free

McGill-Queen's University Press acknowledges the support of the
Canada Council for the Arts for our publishing program. We also
acknowledge the financial support of the Government of Canada
through the Book Publishing Industry Development Program
(BPIDP) for our publishing activities.

Library and Archives Canada Cataloguing in Publication

Tuberculosis then and now : perspectives on the history of an
infectious disease / edited by Flurin Condrau and Michael Worboys.

(McGill-Queen's/Associated Medical Services studies in the history
of medicine, health, and society 35)
Includes index.
ISBN 978-0-7735-3600-5 (bnd)
ISBN 978-0-7735-3601-2 (pbk)

1. Tuberculosis. 2. Tuberculosis – History. I. Condrau, Flurin
II. Worboys, Michael, 1948– III. Series: McGill-Queen's/Associated
Medical Services studies in the history of medicine, health, and
society 35

RC311.T86 2010   616.9'95   C2009-905281-4

Typeset by Jay Tee Graphics Ltd. in 10.5/13 Sabon

Contents

TUBERCULOSIS THEN AND NOW

upward" march of medical science. Medical sociology, the social sciences, and social history affected the writing of medical history only in the second half of the twentieth century. Burnham wrote of the continuing tensions between what he loosely defined as the PhDs and the MDs in the writing of medical history.[3] This characterisation is perhaps somewhat misleading for the history of medicine as a whole, especially in ignoring the richness of the work of pioneers such as Fielding H. Garrison, Henry Sigerist, and Erwin Ackerknecht, amongst others; however, it is useful for delineating approaches to writing the history of tuberculosis.[4]

In 1925 Dr Lawrence F. Flick, the founder of the Pennsylvania Society for the Prevention of Tuberculosis and medical director of the Henry Phipps Institute for the Prevention and Study of Tuberculosis published *Development of Our Knowledge of Tuberculosis*. He introduced his history with these words: "Now that it [tuberculosis] is understood, and its mysteries cleared up, and the way paved for its extermination, the story of how this was done is of gripping interest."[5] In 1949 S. Lyle Cummins, formerly professor of tuberculosis in the Welsh National School of Medicine and director of research for a Welsh anti-tuberculosis organization, published *Tuberculosis in History: From the Seventeenth Century to Our Own Times*. He concluded his history with Robert Koch's discovery of the tubercle bacillus in 1882, explaining, "For us, his conquest of tuberculosis is enough! We stand forever his debtors for this wonderful clearing of the way which has brought the light of truth to bear on the dark and devious journey on which we are bent."[6] For others the climax came later. Selman Waksman, professor of microbiology at Rutgers University, who is credited with the isolation of streptomycin, the first modern anti-tuberculosis drug, in 1943, published a history of tuberculosis in 1964 called *The Conquest of Tuberculosis*.[7] Concluding the section from ancient times until 1943, he explained, "This completes the story of tuberculosis until 1943. Then the picture looked gloomy indeed."[8] He then proceeded to describe the successes of chemotherapy. In his story true progress thus came at a later date, but he nevertheless set up a model of the advance of medical science in opposition to the ignorance that preceded it. Sometimes the account was more directly autobiographical, such as that by W.A. Murray, a Scottish tuberculosis sanatorium medical superintendent. In 1981 he published *A Life Worth Living: Fifty Years in Medicine,* in which he explained,

"When the life of the writer coincides with one of the greatest successes in the defeat of a widespread killing disease, and he played a significant part in that defeat, his theme becomes irresistible."[9]

Invoking similar motives of unmitigated success, George Jasper Wherret, entitled his book *The Miracle of Empty Beds*.[10] A more recent example of this genre is *Pioneers in Medicine and Their Impact on Tuberculosis* by Thomas Daniel, professor emeritus of medicine and international health at Case Western Reserve University, Cleveland, Ohio. This volume presents a series of short biographical accounts of six men Daniel describes as "unrestrainable geniuses" in the ways in which they helped to "conquer" tuberculosis through their respective contributions to pathology, bacteriology, public health, immunology, epidemiology, and antibiotics.[11] During the two centuries spanning the lives of these men, he explained, "the medicine we know today emerged from the chrysalis of mysticism and metamorphosed into an evidence-based discipline."[12]

Burnham wrote that much "traditional" medical history was about using the past to establish an identity, with doctors addressing fellow doctors. This applied to all the authors cited above. Daniel explained that he was inspired to write this history after almost four decades of personal involvement in chest diseases. His target audience, he claimed, consisted of "physicians, biomedical scientists, and other health professionals who are my present and future colleagues in the crusade to conquer tuberculosis [and who] will likely find that knowledge of their intellectual origins enriches their present science and art."[13] Firmly equating knowledge with control, Daniel expressed his belief that thinking about those origins "will help us achieve the new insights needed for further conquests."[14] He did not attempt to contextualise, deconstruct, or unravel the scientific discourses he described.

As noted above, different approaches were being practised by other historians. Henry Sigerist, who was at the Johns Hopkins University, Baltimore, wrote of tuberculosis as "an extremely social disease," but did not develop this insight.[15] René Dubos and Jean Dubos also described tuberculosis in their 1952 history as a "social disease" that presented problems that transcended the conventional medical approach. In their view, the destructive powers of the disease were "the consequence of gross defects in social organization, and of errors in individual behaviour."[16] However, they could not entirely escape a progressive view of history, arguing that once the cause of tuberculosis was known, preventive measures "acquired the compelling strength of common sense."[17]

The 1970s saw modern medicine viewed more critically from many directions, but the work of Ivan Illich was particularly influential. Illich began his book *Limits to Medicine* with the words, "the medical establishment has become a major threat to health," and set out how iatrogenesis – physician-caused illness – was evident in clinical medicine and in the wider medicalisation of everyday life.[18] Interestingly, many of his examples of clinical iatrogenesis were drawn from René Dubos's *Mirage of Medicine* and concerned the emergence of antibiotic-resistant bacteria, which had been a problem with the treatment of tuberculosis since the first use of streptomycin. Such critiques inspired new approaches to the history of medicine, including the history of tuberculosis. An influential work was Susan Sontag's *Illness as Metaphor*.[19] Relying heavily on Dubos's history, Sontag's writing helped promote explorations of the many meanings of the experience of the disease by individuals and different groups, within and without medicine.

Another profound influence on the new social history of medicine emerged from the work of Thomas McKeown, professor of social medicine at Birmingham University, who published *The Modern Rise of Population* and *The Role of Medicine*, based on research that he had carried out over the course of the previous decades.[20] His work has been described as "something of a conceptual revolution in the disciplines of history and medicine, overturning a long-standing general orthodoxy regarding the importance of medical science and the medical profession in bringing about the decline in mortality which accompanied industrialization in Britain."[21] Analysing Britain's death records from 1838, McKeown argued that advances in medicine played a minor role in the historic decline of mortality and instead pointed to improvements in the standard of living as the main factor. He showed that death rates from the major killer diseases had already declined dramatically before modern innovations in the form of chemotherapy and immunisation. Tuberculosis was central to his thesis – the steady decline in the disease's mortality could be tracked from mid-nineteenth century; immunisation and chemotherapy were not introduced until after 1940, by which time mortality rates were a tenth of their level in 1838. McKeown challenged an important feature of the medical profession's claim to prestige and suggested that the actions of individual doctors had contributed little to the long-term decline in mortality.

In 1970 Thomas McKeown's Inaugural Lecture of the Society for the Social History of Medicine (SSHM) asserted that "the social history of medicine must be medical history with the 'public interest' put in."[22] A later president of the society, Charles Webster, urged in 1976 "relegating to a subordinate place any linear account of medical progress, in favour of an approach which is primarily concerned with contributing to an understanding of the dynamics of any particular society."[23] The birth of the SSHM heralded new approaches within medical history, and as early as 1980, Samuel Shortt wrote of the rise of the "new social history of medicine," explaining that the subject was "fundamental to the discipline of social history."[24] The challenges within the new discipline were taken up in relation to tuberculosis by social historians from the 1980s. Reviewing four histories of tuberculosis in 1989, Nancy Tomes wrote of "a remarkable renaissance of interest among scholars in Europe and the United States" in the White Plague. She located this renaissance in the intellectual agenda that had emerged in the 1970s. "In particular," she wrote, "the new work on tuberculosis reflects two aspects of interest in what might loosely be termed the 'social construction of illness,' that is, the interplay between biological and cultural realities in the conception and treatment of disease."[25]

This "remarkable renaissance of interest" was sustained and intensified over the following two decades when more than a dozen monographs were published specifically on tuberculosis, along with many more articles and chapters. Historians have been particularly fond of writing national case studies, linking changing understandings to public health policies and national political, social, and economic developments: Sweden,[26] Britain,[27] France,[28] Germany,[29] Canada,[30] South Africa,[31] Japan,[32] and Austria[33] are just a few countries for which there are now modern histories of tuberculosis. These histories also emphasise the varying ways in which the disease was experienced and constructed differently across time and space.

However, the context for these studies had started to change. In the light of the escalation of tuberculosis cases in conjunction with the HIV/AIDS pandemic, in 1993 the WHO declared tuberculosis a global emergency and emphasised the new level of threat from new multiple drug-resistant strains of the tubercle bacillus. In their book on *The Return of the White Plague*, Matthew Gandy and Alimuddin Zumla declared, "The history of tuberculosis is a story of medical failure."[34]

The chapters in this volume develop these perspectives in two areas: first, in studies of the experiences of patients, the public, and activists with the illness and its treatment; and second, in studies that show the contingent character of anti-tuberculosis policies across time and space.

PATIENT AND PUBLIC EXPERIENCES

One of the goals of the new histories of medicine was to foreground patients, breaking away from the doctor- and science-focused accounts of that had been prominent previously.[35] Because the disease had struck the rich and the famous as well as the poor and nameless and because a romantic image that had allegedly arisen around the disease, patients were not entirely neglected in earlier histories of tuberculosis. Dr J. Harley Williams, long-serving secretary of the National Association for the Prevention of Tuberculosis, whose narrative concerned "the heroic pioneers in the anti-tuberculosis campaign," explained that "the intention of this book is to present tuberculosis not merely as a series of theoretical discoveries and administrative acts, but as a great catalyser in a human being's life."[36] He aimed to achieve this by devoting a chapter to "some of its greatest victims" – John Keats, Frederic Chopin, the Brontës, Robert Louis Stevenson, D.H. Lawrence, Anton Pavlovich Chekov, and Katherine Mansfield. In his 1999 book, consultant pathologist Thomas Dormandy narrated with great style and compassion the sad stories of famous literary and artistic people who had died of tuberculosis. He referred to a thread running through his story, traditionally known as *spes phthisica,* the hope commonly found among sufferers that was described by William Osler as "the Great Delusion." From his accounts of these famous people, Dormandy argued that tuberculosis inspired its many victims to live and fight, and above all to be creative.[37] To what extent the many millions of other sufferers were also inspired to creativity, however, remains unknown.

Social histories of tuberculosis have attempted to reach "ordinary" sufferers from the disease. Barbara Bates did so through analysing correspondence between patients and Dr Lawrence Flick, who had himself suffered from tuberculosis.[38] Sheila Rothman drew upon an impressive list of personal diaries and letters of over one hundred sufferers to weave a social history of the disease in America.[39] Personal narratives involved families, friends, career choices, child rearing, and spiritual experiences. However, historians such as Rothman still struggled to find a wide representation among their subjects. Rothman admitted that Deborah Fiske, the subject of the section of her book on the female "invalid" of the early nineteenth century, was not typical of all women invalids; she was wealthier and better educated than most. Yet Rothman concluded, "In Deborah's life we will see the way consumption affected women's education, marriage, child-rearing practices, female friendship, religious precepts, and relationships with doctors, and how it altered the basic fabric of the community."[40] Did she perhaps read too much into the experiences of this one wealthy educated woman?

In the 1940s, Henry Sigerist drew attention to the importance of studying the "sociology of the patient" in the tuberculosis sanatorium, who was driven by one task, "to recover."[41] Sanatorium experience has been the subject of much modern historical analysis. An influential theoretical basis was provided by Erving Goffman's "total institution" thesis, which explained how residents were "institutionalised" by their experiences in the sanatorium. Patient experience included a subculture within establishments, or a "hospital underlife," though relations between staff and patients were patriarchal.[42] Linda Bryder, Greta Jones, and Flurin Condrau have described the subculture within the tuberculosis sanatoria they researched.[43] Modern histories discussing the relationships between doctors and patients both within and without institutions have argued that patients were not simply victims of a powerful medical profession but rather that they played an active part in negotiating care and treatment.[44] Barron Lerner's study of Firland Sanatorium, Seattle, from 1945 until it closed in 1973, showed its pioneering strategies for controlling one particular sub-set of patients, alcoholic vagrants. Generally regarded as uncooperative, these people had a high rate of discharge from hospital against medical advice, thus limiting the effectiveness of treatment and spreading tuberculosis in the community. From 1949, staff used forcible detention in locked wards for up to twelve months, regardless of a patient's medical condition. Despite this seemingly aggressive policy, Lerner argued that it was not simply an example of the "social control" of a deviant, lower-class population, as there was extensive "negotiation and bargaining" between staff and patients.[45] He contrasted this with modern treatment and argued that the sanatorium did a better job with its clientele than the modern approach of DOT (directly observed therapy), where outpatients take their medications under the direct supervision of an outreach worker. He argued that this was a narrow medical model that did not consider patients' social problems, unless addressing them helped directly improve compliance with the drug regime.

Others too have addressed patients' experiences of the disease and of treatments with an eye to critiquing present-day policies. Katherine Ott explained how nineteenth-century consumption was viewed as a constitutional affliction, one in which the whole body was the site of the disease.[46] Twentieth-century tuberculosis became a technologically based entity, grounded in bacteriology and identified by such tools as tuberculin skin tests, sputum examinations, stethoscope, thermometer, and chest x-rays. The legacy of this recent history for current policy in her view was a total concentration on eradicating the tubercle bacillus, where the tendency to overlook the patient made modern programs and therapeutics highly vulnerable. If germ-directed drugs failed, there were few alternatives. The studies of Richard Coker, Matthew Gandy, and Alimuddin Zumla all pointed out that the very word "non-compliance" implied that the fault lay with the patient.[47] Historians and others have argued for a greater focus on tuberculosis patients' social problems, just as Sigerist did in 1943. The focus on the patients' experiences of the illness and treatment does then have implications for modern approaches to the control of the disease. Rothman enjoined readers in her conclusion to remember that policies to combat any disease profoundly affect individual life chances and life choices. She wrote, "This is finally why it is so important to write the history of disease from the perspective of the patient."[48]

Four chapters in this volume explore the changing and varying experiences of individual patients and the wider public in their encounters with tuberculosis and its treatment. Tim Boon provides an innovative analysis of illness narratives. His particular focus is on tuberculosis films and how they contributed to experiences that were previously largely unknown. Whilst his chapter offers new insights to anyone interested in health education and tuberculosis control, his analysis is particularly important because it reveals previously unknown illness narratives. Boon argues that no history of any disease is ever told without taking into account previous attempts at narration. In other words, it should not come as a surprise that patients, films, and medical science interact in an interesting, yet complex, way to shape a collective experience of illness that then shapes the way the patient narrative is conceptualised.

David Barnes tackles one of the more intriguing cultural features of epidemic diseases, the search for "patient zero" as the initial patient – and origin of infection. His empirical material comes from a recent tuberculosis outbreak in the San Francisco Bay area, but his analysis is most revealing for the understanding of modern epidemics through a complex mixture of motives for the search for patients. What makes Barnes's paper particularly original is its combination of an interest in the culture of acute communicable disease control with an application in chronic diseases, where the proven principle of case detection does not work. As Barnes shows, the epidemiology of tracing the root case becomes a social analysis of tuberculosis, as "patient zero" cases are usually cases involving poor, marginal, or ethnic minorities.

Flurin Condrau's chapter on Erving Goffman and the recent historiography of tuberculosis provides a detailed study of methodological issues in the history of medical institutions. Using Goffman's important theory of the "total institution," Condrau develops empirical criteria to assess the validity of the theory. While he claims that the theory of a total institution is of limited analytical strength, a detailed investigation reveals interesting aspects of sanatoria that have previously been overlooked. In particular, he tackles the long-held view that the sanatorium offered a standardised experience for all patients. Drawing on his own and other authors' empirical work, he reveals a diverse picture of the sanatorium and thereby manages to convey an image of the sanatorium as a multifunctional and multi-dimensional institution that needs to be understood within its local cultural context.

Alison Bashford's account of health immigration policies in Australia over the twentieth century shows how tuberculosis was and remains the central public health concern. The chapter sets out how tuberculosis changed from a domestic disease – *our* disease – to an exotic disease of immigrants – *their* disease. Her chapter demonstrates how Australia's unique position as a new nation of immigrants meant that tuberculosis was always framed in terms of race (indigenous and incoming) and space (keeping out the tuberculous); indeed, in the first decade of the twenty-first century, tuberculosis remains the only condition about which no exceptions are allowed with immigrant visas. Bashford explains how policies evolved with changing patterns of immigration, from predominantly British to wider European and then mainly Asian, and with shifts in medical and popular anxieties, from the Yellow Peril in the late nineteenth century, to the Boat People of the 2000s. Her analysis has to be finely grained to pick up the nuances of nationality, place of origin, religion, and social class; for example, in the case of Britons in the 1950s there were stricter regulations for working class families arriving on assisted passages than for wealthy families on unassisted passages. The narrative is also set against changing immigration laws and practices and the shifts in tuberculosis policy that went with changing medical knowledge and new technologies of management, prevention, and treatment.

Much of the debate on anti-tuberculosis policies continues to be inflected through the debate on Thomas McKeown's thesis, largely because it raises the question of priorities in disease control: should policies be medically based and aim to control the disease or socially focused and aim to promote health. The social histories of tuberculosis by F.B. Smith and Linda Bryder, published in 1988, questioned the role of the anti-tuberculosis campaigns and medical intervention in the decline of tuberculosis in Britain in the nineteenth and twentieth centuries. In her 1989 review, Tomes considered that Smith in particular had been too harsh in his condemnation of the interventions as useless and misguided. She claimed, "historians may fairly question the wisdom of spending money on sanatoria instead of on housing subsidies, but they cannot conclusively prove that the tuberculosis movement as a whole played *no* role in the 'retreat' of the disease. Given this uncertainty over cause and effect, some charity in assessing the public health activities of the past would seem well advised."[49] Flurin Condrau took this further and argued for the historicity of medical success, which implies that sanatorium treatment cannot be measured against modern-day tuberculosis treatments but needs to be understood within a narrative of medical success.[50]

Simon Szreter launched an attack on the McKeown thesis in an influential article in 1988, reinstating some medical contributions to the mortality decline in the form of nineteenth-century public health initiatives, such as sanitation, health education, and housing reform. On the subject of tuberculosis, Szreter admitted that it was probable that the absence of malnutrition in a population was a "necessary condition for the elimination of tuberculosis mortality altogether, [but that it was] equally probable that danger is decreased if other risk factors are reduced: particularly, frequency of incidence of other infectious diseases; but also overcrowding, lack of sunlight, air ventilation and various occupational hazards."[51]

Ongoing debates were not concerned so much with the respective importance of nutrition and housing but rather focused on assessing the relative importance of social conditions versus the role of medical intervention in the form of institutions or targeted public health campaigns. This was the basis of the debate conducted in the pages of the *Social History of Medicine* on events in France. By looking at the continued high death rates from tuberculosis there in the late nineteenth and early twentieth centuries, in comparison to Germany and Britain, Allan Mitchell argued that these high rates resulted from the failure to adopt a coherent and active anti-tuberculosis policy. He concluded, by a form of negative logic, that local sanitary measures and national health reforms were of key importance in reducing deaths from this disease.[52] David Barnes also compared these three nations, but with a focus on their economic history rather than public health systems. All three of the major Western European industrial powers experienced prolonged rises in real wages from 1870 to 1914, but both the real wage levels and their rates of growth differed considerably. France lagged significantly behind the other two and suffered from greater unemployment. In his view this was "another hint that 'standard of living' broadly construed might indeed hold its own as a determinant of France's greater susceptibility to the disease."[53]

Anti-tuberculosis campaigns were the subject of an article on the historical decline of tuberculosis in Europe and America by Leonard Wilson, published in 1991, in which he argued that medical intervention was indeed important in the decline of tuberculosis from the mid-nineteenth century.[54] He attacked both McKeown's thesis on the importance of improving living standards in the decline and Szreter's argument that "the decline of tuberculosis mortality may have been a secondary effect of the decline in other infectious disease brought about by improved water supplies, sanitation, and other public health measures."[55] Wilson responded that "the known cause, means of spread and natural history of tuberculosis in the individual make Szreter's argument improbable, but it is in any case unnecessary because there is another simpler explanation of the historical decline of tuberculosis in England, supported by excellent evidence."[56] This was the effect of placing consumptive patients in workhouses or in Poor Law infirmaries – to separate them from the general populace and to restrict the spread of their infection to others, though this was a "welfare" rather than a medical intervention. According to Wilson, this measure had been set out "with brilliant clarity"[57] by Arthur Newsholme, chief medical officer of the Local Government Board of England and Wales, in *The Prevention of Tuberculosis* (1908). In a response to Wilson's thesis, Linda Bryder pointed out that there was no attempt to segregate tuberculosis cases from other inmates within the Poor Law institutions in the nineteenth century.[58] Discussing tuberculosis in Ireland, Greta Jones commented that "the Irish workhouse, at least before consciousness developed of the need to segregate the tuberculous from other inmates, probably aggravated the problem."[59]

Discussing the institutions set up explicitly for the treatment of tuberculosis, Bryder argued that the patients were in the institutions for only a short proportion of their infective lives: "Exposure to massive doses of the bacillus was of course important, but segregating these people for a few months could not have made much difference."[60] Nor did she accept Wilson's claim that the anti-tuberculosis campaign after 1882 was based on prevention through isolating individuals in institutions. Those who ran tuberculosis sanatoria in the early twentieth century invariably attempted to attract early "curable" cases, rather than advanced cases, who, as Neil McFarlane also noted, often returned home to die.[61] And, as Flurin Condrau observed, patients often went through a series of institutions involving hospitals, poor law infirmaries, and sanatoria at various stages of their illness.[62] Sheila Rothman found in America that many patients left the institutions early, against medical advice, because of the unpleasant conditions there.[63] Barron Lerner too revealed high rates of self-discharge against medical advice at Firland Sanatorium in the early twentieth century.[64] In addition, Flurin Condrau showed in detailed empirical studies that long-term confinement of tuberculosis patients in Britain and Germany was the exception rather than the rule.[65]

Thus, those historians who have researched institutions for tuberculosis and their clientele have provided a different assessment of their efficacy from those relying on the officials like Newsholme, who, as Amy Fairchild and Gerald Oppenheimer observed in 1998, "were not simply neutral commentators but, rather, agents of public health who favored relatively easily engineered targeted interventions ... over politically and technically complex social interventions that would affect a population much wider than infected individuals and their immediate contacts."[66] Richard Coker also noted the debate and concluded that tuberculosis rates had fallen for a variety of reasons, "with improved social conditions (reduced over-crowding, better ventilation, improved nutrition), segregation and the sanatoria movement, and pasteurization all playing a part." Yet he also cited evidence to the effect that "when the majority of the population has already been exposed, isolating even infectious patients may serve little purpose."[67]

While historians question the respective roles of nutrition and other social factors, the most important debates revolve around the relative importance of health intervention in the form of targeted campaigns or medical intervention, on the one hand, and broad-based redistributive social policies, on the other. The specific role of BCG vaccination in tuberculosis control remains contested.[68] Its history has largely been written around the biggest vaccination catastrophe of recent times that claimed the lives of seventy-seven children in the German city of Lübeck in 1931.[69] Further, more fundamental questions about vaccination policy in the light of persisting antivaccinationism still need to be addressed more widely. Writing on recent developments in New York, Coker argued in favour of addressing society's economic and political inequalities in order to achieve long-term control of tuberculosis, an approach that found favour with other social historians such as Georgina Feldberg, Katherine Ott, and Barron Lerner.[70] In their article on the "new" tuberculosis, Gandy and Zumla claimed that the McKeown thesis tended to downplay the politically contested nature of historical outcomes in public health.[71] David Barnes, among others, argued that economic change, on which McKeown placed such emphasis, should be regarded not as a result of "an invisible hand" but as the hard-earned outcome of negotiations and struggles, the result of massive concerted human activity.[72] Szreter pointed out that the McKeown thesis could easily be co-opted by right-wing economists to argue that economic growth, without ameliorating social policies, would control communicable diseases.[73] However, McKeown supporters such as Link and Phelan continued to cite the cherished principle of the importance of social factors in health, or McKeown's "assertion that social conditions are fundamental causes of disease and death."[74]

The debates that have engaged and exercised the minds of historians of tuberculosis, among others, relate to the respective effects of health intervention in the form of targeted campaigns or institutional medical responses and structural social reforms. The question continues in relation to the McKeown thesis: Are public health ends better served by targeted interventions or by broad-based efforts to redistribute the social, political, and economic resources? As Barnes noted in 1991, the debates reflect differing political perspectives.[75] Coker, on the other hand, commenting on tuberculosis being related to poverty, overcrowding, malnutrition, and social inequity, remarked that tuberculosis was "a measure of social justice, hence its fascination."[76] Historians of tuberculosis have engaged in debates that are central not only to the historiography of medicine but to current preventative and curative health policies.

Five chapters in this volume explore the policy issues then and now. John Welshman's analysis of postwar immigration policies and tuberculosis offers insights into the importance of border controls and migration debates. His chapter connects very well with recent historiography on the cultural formation of borders, whilst at the same time tackling tuberculosis-specific regulations in postwar Britain. Welshman argues that historians are only partially correct in arguing that after the Second World War there was a decline in the belief that susceptibility to tuberculosis was dependant on racial factors. Through comparing Irish and South Asian immigrants, he emphasises the continuity of racial stereotypes, to the extent that local public health doctors continued to attribute tuberculosis to a combination of racial weakness, inadequate nutrition, and overcrowding. His view is that tuberculosis debates in postwar Britain remained highly racialised.

Michael Worboys's chapter explores the views of the generation of British doctors before McKeown who first recognised and discussed the long-term fall in tuberculosis mortality. He identifies five groups with distinct explanations of the decline, each of which emphasised a single principal factor. The five groups and their main determinants were the insanitationists, who stressed the role of general sanitary improvements; the infectionists, who looked to the control of person-to-person spread; the hygienists, who pointed to health education and lifestyle changes; the diathesians, who contended that the disease had eliminated the "unfit" who had an inherited susceptibility; and the tubercularisationists, who believed that the population had developed acquired herd immunity. Worboys links the different views with the social position and interests of group members; however, his groups were not exclusive, as some individuals supported more than one position. With this elegant use of ideal types, Worboys also begins to problematise the disease category of tuberculosis, which meant different things to the groups involved. The views of some of the groups can be mapped onto the McKeown debate; however, Worboys highlights two important differences: contemporaries were interested in morbidity as well as mortality, and their views were developed in policy formulation.

Jorge Molero-Mesa explores the political struggle of anti-tuberculosis policies in Restoration Spain between the 1870s and 1930s. He shows how social medicine was developed to improve national efficiency and to reform working class health through the promotion of responsible behaviour. This approach differed from that of nineteenth-century epidemiologists, who had linked the rise in tuberculosis to deteriorating social conditions and the misery of working-class life, and instead focused on the bacillus and halting its spread through changes in individual behaviour. In Spain the anti-tuberculosis movement favoured establishing dispensaries rather than sanatoria and sought to raise consciousness and funds through a national tuberculosis day, which was symbolised by a flower symbol. In opposition, socialist organizations established Red Flower Day, during which they called for improved wages and conditions. This alternative campaign was extended to the view that workers had the right not to have tuberculosis and to the politicisation of health more widely. This became a pivotal moment in the history of the left in Spain; indeed, the main symbol of the left in Spain continues to be the Red Flower.

Peter Atkins's chapter on the history of bovine tuberculosis in interwar Britain draws on an innovative methodological approach to explain the scientific and political debates around bovine tuberculosis. Inspired by recent political and social theory, Atkins applies concepts such as an inside/outside model of government and policy development, alongside actor-network theory, to analyse the slow and tortuous progress of policy-making on bovine tuberculosis in Britain in the first half of the twentieth century. The struggle between radical and conservative forces was visible at all levels of the food chain, but Atkins's argument emphasises the voices of selected individuals as representatives of views expressed inside and outside Westminster and Whitehall.

Helen Valier's contribution tackles the collaborative antibiotics trials in India in the 1950s. Valier contributes to a recent wave of studies of the arrival and development of modern chemotherapy against tuberculosis. The 1950s were a remarkable period, for the arrival of demonstrably effective antibiotic therapies fundamentally changed the way the disease was defined, perceived, treated, experienced, and ultimately survived. Nevertheless, this was also a decade of renewed international collaboration in disease control, and the chemotherapy trials organized in Madras and Bangalore were part of the wider development of international cooperation in health care in a post-imperialist world. As Valier shows, the partners in this particular cooperation all pursued a range of interests, linking Britain's Medical Research Council, whose agenda was shaped by the domestic policies of the NHS, with international issues.

As well as individually covering novel subject matter in the history of tuberculosis, together the essays in this volume also bring new methodological and theoretical perspectives that will both enliven and deepen the history of the disease. Our authors make use of novel sources; they use old and new theories, from Weber through Goffman to Latour; they link class, race, and politics; and they show the changing constitution of public health spaces and their boundaries. We are equally pleased to see all authors, either directly or indirectly, speak to current policy issues, specifically with regard to tuberculosis, but we hope also to other communicable diseases.

NOTES

1 John Bunyan, *The Life and Death of Mr Badman* (1680; Oxford: Oxford University Press 1980), 148.

2 Throughout this introduction we have used the word "tuberculosis" to refer to "pulmonary tuberculosis" and have avoided the abbreviation TB,

as this is confusingly used for both the disease – tuberculosis – and its necessary causative agent – the tubercle bacillus.

3 John C. Burnham, "Garrison Lecture: How the Concept of Profession Evolved in the Work of Historians of Medicine," *Bulletin of the History of Medicine* 70, 1 (1996): 1–24.

4 Frank Huisman and John Harley Warner, "Medical Histories," in Frank Huisman and John Harley Warner (eds.), *Locating Medical History: The Stories and Their Meanings* (Baltimore: Johns Hopkins University Press 2006), 1–32.

5 Lawrence F. Flick, *Development of Our Knowledge of Tuberculosis* (Philadelphia: Author 1925), preface.

6 S. Lyle Cummins, *Tuberculosis in History: From the Seventeenth Century to Our Own Times* (London: Balliere, Tindall & Cox 1949), 198.

7 A recent summary of the controversy over the "discovery" of streptomycin is given in Thomas M. Daniel, "Selman Abraham Waksman and the Discovery of Streptomycin," *International Journal of Tuberculosis and Lung Disease* 9, 2 (2005): 120–2.

8 Selman A. Waksman, *The Conquest of Tuberculosis* (Berkeley: University of California Press 1964), 100.

9 W.A. Murray, *A Life Worth Living: Fifty Years in Medicine* (Haddington: Author 1982), preface. In the same tradition was a 1978 history by a British chest physician, Robert Young Keers: Robert Y. Keers, *Pulmonary Tuberculosis: A Journey down the Centuries,* (London: Bailliere Tindall 1978).

10 George J. Wherrett, *The Miracle of the Empty Beds: A History of Tuberculosis in Canada* (Toronto: University of Toronto Press 1977).

11 Thomas M. Daniel, *Pioneers in Medicine and Their Impact on Tuberculosis* (New York: University of Rochester Press 2000), 209.

12 Ibid., xi.

13 Ibid., xii.

14 Ibid., 33.

15 Henry E. Sigerist, *Civilization and Disease* (1st ed., Cornell University 1943, reprint Chicago: The University of Chicago Press 1962), 81.

16 René Dubos and Jean Dubos, *The White Plague: Tuberculosis, Man and Society* (Boston: Little, Brown and Company 1952, reprint with a foreword by David Mechanic and an introductory essay by Barbara Gutmann Rosenkrantz, New Brunswick: Rutgers 1987), xxxviii.

17 Ibid., 172.

18 Ivan Illich, *Limits to Medicine: Medical Nemesis, the Expropriation of Health* (New York: Harmondsworth 1977).

19 Susan Sontag, *Illness as Metaphor* (New York: Farrar, Straus & Giroux 1977).

20 Thomas McKeown, *The Modern Rise of Population* (London: Edward Arnold 1976); Thomas McKeown, *The Role of Medicine: Dream, Mirage, or Nemesis?* (London: Nuffield Provincial Hospitals Trust 1976).

21 Simon Szreter, "The Importance of Social Intervention in Britain's Mortality Decline, c.1850–1914: A Re-interpretation of the Role of Public Health," *Social History of Medicine* 1, 1 (1988): 2.

22 Webster cited in Dorothy Porter, "The Mission of Social History of Medicine: An Historical View," *Social History of Medicine* 8, 3 (1995): 348.

23 Ibid., 351.

24 Samuel Shortt, "The New Social History of Medicine: Some Implications for Research," *Archivaria*, 10 (1980): 5–22.

25 Nancy J. Tomes, "The White Plague Revisited: Essay Review," *Bulletin of the History of Medicine* 63 (1989): 467. The four histories were Linda Bryder, *Below the Magic Mountain: A Social History of Tuberculosis in Twentieth-Century Britain* (Oxford: Clarendon Press 1988); F.B. Smith, *The Retreat of Tuberculosis, 1850–1950* (London: Croom Helm 1988); Michael E. Teller, *The Tuberculosis Movement: A Public Health Campaign in the Progressive Era* (Westport, CT: Greenwood Press 1988), and the 1987 reprint Dubos, *The White Plague.*

26 Britt-Inger Puranen, *Tuberkulos: En sjukdoms förekomst och dess orsaker, Sverige 1750–1980* (Umea: Umea Universitet Förlag 1984).

27 Bryder, *Below the Magic Mountain*; Smith, *The Retreat of Tuberculosis.*

28 Pierre Guillaume, *Du Déséspoir au Salut: Les Tuberculeux aux 19e et 20e Siècles* (Paris: Aubier 1986); Dominique Dessertine and Olivier Faure, *Combattre la tuberculose, 1900–1940* (Lyon: Presses universitaires de Lyon 1988); David S. Barnes, *The Making of a Social Disease: Tuberculosis in Nineteenth-Century France* (Berkeley: University of California Press 1995).

29 Flurin Condrau, *Lungenheilanstalt und Patientenschicksal: Sozialgeschichte der Tuberkulose in Deutschland und England im späten 19. und frühen 20. Jahrhundert* (Göttingen: Vandenhoeck & Ruprecht 2000); Sylvelyn Hähner-Rombach, *Sozialgeschichte der Tuberkulose: Vom Kaiserreich bis zum Ende des Zweiten Weltkriegs unter besonderer Berücksichtigung Württembergs* (Stuttgart: Steiner 2000).

30 Katherine McCuaig, *The Weariness, the Fever, and the Fret: The Campaign against Tuberculosis in Canada, 1900–1950* (Montreal: McGill-Queen's University Press 1999).

31 Randall M. Packard, *White Plague, Black Labor: Tuberculosis and the Political Economy of Health and Disease in South Africa* (Berkeley: University of California Press 1989).

32 William Johnston, *The Modern Epidemic: A History of Tuberculosis in Japan* (Cambridge: Harvard University Press 1995); Mahito Fukuda, *Kekkaku no Bunkashi* [Cultural History of Tuberculosis in Japan] (Nagoya 1995).

33 Elisabeth Dietrich-Daum, *Die "Wiener Krankheit": Eine Sozialgeschichte der Tuberkulose in Osterreich* (Vienna: Verlag für Geschichte und Politik 2007).

34 Alimuddin Zumla and Matthew Gandy, "Epilogue: Politics, Science and the 'New' Tuberculosis," in Matthew Gandy and Alimuddin Zumla (eds.), *The Return of the White Plague: Global Poverty and the "New" Tuberculosis* (London: Verso 2003), 237.

35 Flurin Condrau, "The Patient's View Meets the Clinical Gaze," *Social History of Medicine* 20, 3 (2007): 225–40.

36 J. Harley Williams, *Requiem for a Great Killer: The Story of Tuberculosis* (London: Health Horizon 1973), 125, 14.

37 Thomas Dormandy, *The White Death: A History of Tuberculosis* (London: The Hambledon Press 1999), 392.

38 Barbara Bates, *Bargaining for Life: A Social History of Tuberculosis, 1876–1938* (Philadelphia: University of Pensylvania Press 1992).

39 Sheila M. Rothman, *Living in the Shadow of Death: Tuberculosis and the Social Experience of Illness in American History* (New York: Basic Books 1994), 252.

40 Ibid., 79.

41 Sigerist, *Civilization and Disease,* 80.

42 Erving Goffman, *Asylums: Essays on the Social Situation of Mental Patients and Other Inmates* (Garden City, NY: Anchor Books 1961).

43 Bryder, *Below the Magic Mountain,* 199–226; Greta Jones, *"Captain of All These Men of Death": The History of Tuberculosis in Nineteenth and Twentieth Century Ireland* (Amsterdam: Rodopi 2001), 159–85; Flurin Condrau, "Who Is the Captain of All These Men of Death? The Social Structure of Tuberculosis Sanatorium Patients in Postwar Germany," *Journal of Interdisciplinary History* 32, 2 (2001): 243–62.

44 Bates, *Bargaining for Life,* 59, 330; Bryder, *Below the Magic Mountain,* 179–82; Katherine Ott, *Fevered Lives: Tuberculosis in American Culture since 1870* (Cambridge, MA: Harvard University Press 1996), 153.

45 Lerner, *Contagion and Confinement,* 8.

46 Ott, *Fevered Lives,* 165–6.

47 Richard J. Coker, *From Chaos to Coercion: Detection and the Control of Tuberculosis* (New York: St Martin's Press 2000); Matthew Gandy and Alimuddin Zumla, "The Resurgence of Disease: Social and Historical Perspectives on the 'New' Tuberculosis," *Social Science and Medicine* 55, 5 (2002): 389.

48 Rothman, *Living in the Shadow of Death,* 252.

49 Tomes, "The White Plague Revisited," 477.

50 Flurin Condrau, "Urban Tuberculosis Patients and Sanatorium Treatment in the Early Twentieth Century," in Anne Borsay Peter Shapely (eds.), *Medicine, Charity and Mutual Aid: The Consumption of Health and Welfare, c.1550–1950* (Aldershot: Ashgate 2007), 183–206.

51 Szreter, "The Importance of Social Intervention," 13.

52 Allan Mitchell, "An Inexact Science: The Statistics of Tuberculosis in Late Nineteenth-Century France," *Social History of Medicine* 3, 3 (1990):387–403.

53 David S. Barnes, "The Rise and Fall of Tuberculosis in Belle-Epoque France: A Reply to Allan Mitchell," *Social History of Medicine* 5, 2 (1992):287. See also Barnes, *The Making of a Social Disease.*

54 Leonard G. Wilson, "The Historical Decline of Tuberculosis in Europe and America: Its Causes and Significance," *Journal of the History of Medicine and Allied Sciences* 45, 3 (1990): 366–96.

55 Ibid., 372.

56 Ibid.

57 Ibid.

58 Linda Bryder, "Comments on 'The Historical Decline of Tuberculosis in Europe and America: Its Causes and Significance,'" correspondence, *Journal of the History of Medicine* 46, 3 (1991):358–68.

59 Jones, *Captain of All These Men of Death,* 45.

60 Bryder, "Comments on 'The Historical Decline of Tuberculosis,'" 359.

61 McFarlane, "Hospitals, Housing and Tuberculosis in Glasgow," 70.

62 Flurin Condrau, "The Institutional Career of Tuberculosis Patients in Britain and Germany," in John Henderson and Peregrine Horden (eds.), *The Impact of Hospitals in Europe, 1000–2002* (Oxford: Peter Lang 2007), 327–57.

63 Rothman, *Living in the Shadow of Death,* 209.

64 Lerner, *Contagion and Confinement,* 29.

65 Condrau, *Lungenheilanstalt und Patientenschicksal.*

66 Amy L. Fairchild and Gerald M. Oppenheimer, "Public Health Nihilism vs Pragmatism: History, Politics, and the Control of Tuberculosis,"

American Journal of Public Health 88, 7 (1998): 1105–18; Paul Farmer and Edward Nardell, "Editorial," *American Journal of Public Health* 88, 7 (1998):1014–16.

67 Coker, *From Chaos to Coercion*, 148–9.

68 See Georgina D. Feldberg, *Disease and Class: Tuberculosis and the Shaping of Modern North American Society* (New Brunswick: Rutgers University Press 1995); Linda Bryder, "'We Shall Not Find Salvation in Inoculation': BCG Vaccination in Scandinavia, Britain and the USA, 1921–1960," *Social Science and Medicine* 49, 9 (1999): 1157–67.

69 Christian Bonah, "Le drame de Lübeck: La vaccination BCG, le procès Calmette et les Richtlinien de 1931," in Christian Bonah, Etienne Lépicard, and Volker Roelcke (eds.), La *Médecine expérimentale au tribunal: Implications éthiques de quelques procès médicaux du XXe siècle européen* (Paris: Editions des Archives Contemporaines 2003), 65–94.

70 Coker, *From Chaos to Coercion;* Feldberg, *Disease and Class;* Ott, *Fevered Lives;* Lerner, *Contagion and Confinement;* Lerner, "New York City's Tuberculosis Control Efforts," 758.

71 Gandy and Zumla, "The Resurgence of Disease," 389.

72 Barnes, "The Rise and Fall," 289.

73 Simon Szreter, "The McKeown Thesis, Rethinking McKeown: The Relationship between Public Health and Social Change," *American Journal of Public Health* 92, 5 (2002): 723.

74 Bruce G. Link and Jo C. Phelan, "McKeown and the Idea that Social Conditions are Fundamental Causes of Disease," *American Journal of Public Health* 92, 5 (2002): 730–2; see also Bernard Harris, "Public Health, Nutrition and the Decline of Mortality: The McKeown Debate Revisited," *Social History of Medicine* 17, 3 (2004): 379–407.

75 Barnes, "The Rise and Fall of Tuberculosis," 289–90.

76 Coker, *From Chaos to Coercion*, 209.

2

Lay Disease Narratives, Tuberculosis, and Health Education Films

TIM BOON

INTRODUCTION

This essay makes a speculative proposal: by using an approach to tuberculosis that focuses on the storied nature of lay understandings of disease, it may be possible to gain a broad grasp of its place in the culture of the past. It is a contribution to the strand within medical history that seeks to move beyond the social historical towards the cultural historical in an attempt to make an account of the past that places the experience of disease and medicine proportionally as an aspect of life and not its whole. Because the prevalence and threat of tuberculosis have declined so markedly, especially in the West, older historical accounts have often tended to acquire teleological underpinnings, as the titles of its histories denote, whether *Requiem for a Great Killer* or *The Retreat of Tuberculosis*. The metaphors may have been liturgical or military, but the story was essentially one of medical interventions and their progress against a bacterium or of social and economic change effecting the same result.[1] Social historical scholarship, including that of Lynda Bryder, Sheila Rothman, and Katherine Ott, has drawn a richer picture, especially as regards how the disease was experienced by patients.[2] This essay builds on this more recent historiography to propose a view of tuberculosis that addresses its *cultural* presence, the variety of beliefs – held not only by those suffering or treating the disease but by the whole of society – in the culture of particular periods.

It is certain that diseases have an incalculably large presence in culture, for the healthy as much as for the diseased. This essay proposes that such a cultural presence may be understood by adopting an approach – extrapolated from the studies of scholars including Paul Ricoeur and Paul Cobley – that stresses the primacy of narration. Tuberculosis, because of its long historical prevalence, provides particularly good ground to assess this narrative approach. But if it is of value here, it clearly also has much broader applicability to other diseases. Susan Sontag has suggested that "everyone who is born holds dual citizenship, in the kingdom of the well and in the kingdom of the sick. Although we all prefer only to use the good passport, sooner or later each of us is obliged, at least for a spell, to identify ourselves as citizens of that other place."[3] But for most of us, for most of the time, the other country of serious disease is like L.P. Hartley's past, a foreign country where people do things differently. If Sontag's dual citizenship metaphor is to stand, we must accept not only that we are daily crossing in our imaginations the border between the states of health and illness but that the border is broad. We may say that it is narratives that propel us in that borderland.

The beliefs of *patients* have received enhanced attention in both history of medicine and medical practice in recent decades. Historians of medicine pursuing the implications of the postwar turn to the social have, since the 1980s, placed an enhanced stress on patients' experience.[4] The two half-generation-old canonical texts on the history of tuberculosis, Bryder's *Below the Magic Mountain* and Smith's *The Retreat of Tuberculosis*, in their different ways both incorporate the patient's view of this particular disease, a historiographical tendency continued and impressively deepened in the work of Rothman and Ott. Rothman, in particular, stresses what she calls "patient narratives," but she means the term as a synonym for "patient accounts," rather than the meaning employed in the current essay, that the storied nature of lay disease accounts is relevant to our understanding of the cultural history of disease. The significance to *medical practice* of patients' narratives of disease was marked by the appearance of Howard Brodie's *Stories of Sickness* (1987) and Greenhalgh and Hurwitz's collection *Narrative Based Medicine* (1998). In this latter example of medicine's own linguistic turn, they argue that a more effective clinical practice could result from doctors paying greater attention to patient narratives. As they say, "The clinical experience of health professionals ... demonstrates that episodes of sickness are, if nothing else, important milestones in the enacted narratives of patients' lives."[5] This pattern, in its turn, can be traced to the psychologisation of general practice instigated by Michael Balint from the 1950s.[6]

This contribution looks beyond patients at the broader category of lay people, those not – or not yet – numbered amongst the sick. It is concerned with a slightly different aspect, the *possibility* that we may be sick, or may become so, and that this possibility may also be understood using a narrative-focussed approach. That is to say, the ostensibly well carry within them narratives of sickness and health. As sociologists of health and illness have shown, people in general constantly experience symptoms, but it is comparatively rarely that they get as far as reporting illness at a doctor's surgery. In the "hierarchy of resort" model, many symptoms will be treated with aspirin or a night's sleep, and only in more severe cases will individuals resort to medical opinions and intervention.[7] I wish to suggest here that a narrative approach to tuberculosis promises a way of discussing what the ostensibly well may have believed about serious disease.

The first half of this chapter presents the arguments of some of those who have worked on narrative and sees how these arguments might apply in the case of tuberculosis, both in the clinic and for lay people, before focussing more particularly on the wide range of tuberculosis stories in British culture beyond mainstream medicine. I argue in the second half of the chapter that the narrative approach has particular potential in relation to health education. Where a modern social historian might be interested in the reception and impact of health education, the few historical studies devoted to the subject have tended to be limited to the production of campaigns, paper materials, and films.[8] This focus is only partially the product of historiographical preference, as evidence of reception is thin on the ground, and, even if one's preferences are empirical, it is necessary to adopt various theoretical approaches to gain access to audience experience.[9] The potential of the narrative approach is to see the occasions on which members of the laity experienced health education as moments of interaction between their pre-existing narratives and narratives that medical and state authorities were seeking to impose. It provides a language for describing why the laity might not simply have adopted the dominant medical discourses about tuberculosis and other diseases.

NARRATIVES IN LITERATURE, CINEMA, AND LIFE

In various ways, writers on narrative speak of the different components of storytelling: narrative, story, plot, sequence, space, time. Narrative, according to Paul Ricoeur, links human perception and the passage of time: "time becomes human to the extent that it is articulated through a narrative mode, and narrative attains its full meaning when it becomes a condition of temporal existence."[10] In the specific terms used by narratologists, "story" is the set of events that may be represented in any narrative, and these events have their own literal time sequence. "Narrative" is the conveying of the events in the story, not necessarily in the same sequence. Where there is a chain of causation that connects the events in the narrative, this chain is known as "plot." Many narratives may be made from a single story. But the narrator places these events in a sequence that serves the context of use. "All narratives," as Paul Cobley says, "are the movement from a beginning point to a finishing point ... [But even] the most crude and flimsy narratives must have something between their beginnings and ends ... Narrative must entail some kind of delay or even diversions, detours and digressions." And again: "Representational systems such as narrative work to facilitate the recognition of such phenomena as sequence and causality. They facilitate the meaningful relations that will transpire with human input."[11]

It is clear that narratives, whilst they are often found in outward cultural works such as novels or films, may also be inward, culture-suffused, ways of thinking about life experience. Narrative theorists assert that storytelling is a definitive human activity. In Cobley's words, "Wherever there are humans there appear to be stories. It is true that people tell stories about life history and about their psyches; people read stories when they consume various media ... and, even when thinking about the world in an 'objective' fashion, scientifically or ethically, the tendency to 'storify' remains."[12] In this view, narratives exist on the stage, on the page, on the screen, in the mind. When they pass from the mind in the form of one of these media, they are conveyed in one of two main modes; either by showing (also known as *mimesis*) or by telling (*diegesis*). Showing is the mode where a story is acted out. Telling is conveyed by a third-person narrator. But in literature there are modes intermediate between showing and telling. Principal amongst these is the "free indirect mode," in which first-person subjectivity is conveyed in third-person form. As David Lodge explains, an example of quoted speech combined with a narrator's description might be "'Is that the clock striking twelve?' Cinderella exclaimed. 'Dear me, I shall be late.'" By contrast, "'Was that the clock striking twelve? She would be late' is free indirect speech."[13] In Lodge's view, the free indirect mode gives the reader access to the subjective experience of characters and authors.

TUBERCULOSIS NARRATIVES

If we follow Cobley's contention about the tendency for people to storify their experience, then we must also accept that the origins of narratives about the life course – about birth, life, disease, and death – are inevitably highly diverse. To open up the question of the sources of such narratives as they touch tuberculosis is one of the aims of this chapter. Narratives about tuberculosis may be told by doctors, by patients, or more broadly in culture. Doctors' narratives – those described by Stuart Hogarth and Lara Marks as "Golden narratives" – most often use the diegetic, or telling, mode, as is the case with the example I use here, Trousseau's *Lectures in Clinical Medicine*, an 1868 textbook of clinical pathology. This example mingles a clinical case history with a tragic narrative worthy of a romantic novel.[14] "GENTLEMEN: – You have seen in bed 5, St Bernard's ward, a young woman between twenty-four and twenty-five years of age, the subject of *rapid* phthisis ... This young woman was confined on the 14th March ... upon several occasions, I interrogated her regarding her antecedents, with a view to discover whether she has any previous symptoms of chest disease." At this point, he begins to slip into free indirect mode; it is as though you hear her voice conveyed when he says that, "she replied that no one was less subject to catarrhal affections of the chest than she was. She said that from time to time, she had colds in her head, but had never had cough ... on the 23rd of last March – five weeks ago – she began to cough. From the first, her cough was severe, though it could not be called very violent. Not being able by any means to get rid of it, she resolved to come into the hospital." Finally, with some discussion of clinical signs, he returns to the simple telling, or diegetic, model: "Thus, an opportunity was afforded of being present to witness the advance of the disease ... It was only too evident that ... phthisis progressing with fearful rapidity was threatening to carry off this young woman in a very brief space of time – perhaps in two months, in six weeks, or even sooner."[15]

In the free indirect passage we experience the young woman's internal narrative. First the cough, then the cough that stays, then the hospital visit. Did she suspect tuberculosis? We cannot tell. But lay peoples' tuberculosis narratives often have such plotted chains of events. H.D. Chalke, for example, has commented that "Dylan Thomas ... did not suffer from tuberculosis, but ... he imagined he did; a belief which may have served as an excuse for his alcoholism."[16] The sick man may have disappeared from medical narratives, as Jewson suggested a generation ago, but it is inconceivable that illness narratives disappeared from lay lives.[17] It is possible to perceive an individual's narrative behind those described by writers on tuberculosis. For example, J.R. Bignall's history of Frimley sanatorium describes a group of four patients first discharged in 1905: "The fourth was a dock labourer of thirty-six with six children, also treated like the others with ordinary exercise. His treatment was more successful for he worked as a coppersmith until 1924 and did not lose a day's work. Then he became ill again and lost his job. When he recovered again he was able to get another job making concrete bricks. Four years later he relapsed once more and this time did not recover. He died in July 1930."[18] As with Trousseau, we read this as free indirect mode conveying the life story of the tubercular former dock labourer with a hint of his voice behind its third-person narration. His narrative is formed from the events: losing and gaining employment in cycles governed by recurrence of the disease. There is clear plotting in the leap from diagnosis to social consequence. The narrative resonates with a wide range of stories available in culture, not just about illness, disease, and medicine but about their social consequences. It seems clear then, despite the skepticism of scholars, including Galen Strawson, about the universality of self-narrativisation, that the fear of major disease may fairly be described in narrative terms.[19]

Studies of the audiences for cultural products in the past often founder on the rock of absence of evidence for how paintings, books, films, and other works were received. Michael Baxandall's *Painting and Experience in Fifteenth Century Italy* proposes a way of speaking generically about cultural reception; it suggests the types of ways of seeing possessed by the audiences in the past for whom cultural products were intended. He argues that they may be considered to have possessed a "period eye" – in his study, for example, knowledge of the high price of blue pigment affected how they saw representations of the Virgin Mary; or in another example, experience of using and buying horses made contemporaries' appreciation of how these animals were depicted in paintings much richer than that of most modern viewers.[20] Here I make a similar suggestion: just as viewers of visual works possessed a "period eye," so they also knew a "period storybook," generic within their era, about the life course; about births, about relationships with others, about sickness and death. Approaching the cultural presence of tuberculosis in this way – as one of a set of life narratives – provides a means to generalise about lay beliefs, to talk of the ways in which it was perceived.

TUBERCULOSIS NARRATIVES IN MEDICINE, IRREGULAR MEDICINE, AND CULTURE

It is clear that multiple stories about tuberculosis did exist in interwar culture. Before effective drug therapies, the range of medical stories was diverse. What therapy would have the best effect: work therapy or "hardening-up" in Alpine resorts? Or would collapsing lungs or gold therapy positively resolve the life stories of those who succumbed to the disease? Where medical narratives erupted in public as news stories, they may well have served to challenge, confound, or reinforce individuals' stories. Lay narratives, I propose, were even more diverse than those that orthodox medicine provided. For example, the laity were exposed to the claims of promoters of irregular therapies, including vibromassage, electrotherapy, and herbalism. J.G. Macaura proposed that a mixture of fresh air and use of his patent mechanical massage device, the Macaura "blood circulator," could treat "incipient consumption." He suggested, "treat not too heavily on the abdomen and the backs of legs, then, as patient's strength is being restored, mild treatment may be applied to the spine."[21] Both the expression "incipient consumption" and the temporal phrase "as patient's strength is being restored" are narrative components. We may see all therapeutic interventions as narrative; they propose a world in which the patient will pass through treatment to cure. So, for instance, the proprietors of the Rogers Violet Ray Vitalator argued that "Ozone is especially effective in consumption ... the air of the patient's room must be thoroughly ozonised, so that he or she is getting a suitable amount in the air they breathe."[22] Buried in a general salutary prescription is the implication of cure, of moving on from disease.

Some practitioners also worked within more explicit narrative structures. Take, for example, Professor J.B. Keswick, "the renowned phrenologist and herb specialist," who described three forms of consumption in essentially narrative terms. The description of the third, for example, runs: "In this case there is neither cough nor expectoration at the beginning. There is weakness and a good-for-nothing feeling always present. The least exertion seems to tire the patient. There is a gradual loss of flesh, and weakness increases. After time a slight cough is noticed in the mornings, which grows worse as the weakness increases. The eyes assume an unnatural brilliancy, and the face is flushed towards evening."[23] Under the heading "fast drifting into consumption" a testimonial by "A.C." of Bournemouth published in Keswick's book responded in equally storied form: "Respected Sir, – I feel it my duty, after feeling so much better through your treatment, to write and tell you so. If I had not listened to you I do not know how I should have been by now. My feet, too, are very much better after using the lotion you sent me. I still take the Charcoal, and mother takes it also, and says it keeps her from having the doctor. I scarcely know how to express my sincere thanks to you for making me look and feel what I am. I think it is likely I should have gone into consumption." Both by means of the many editions of his *Herbal Family Guide* – 1s.6d in 1935 – and through his tireless lecturing over fifty years, the lay public, troubled by the possibility of incipient consumption, could indulge in an alternative narrative to that of the sanatorium. This too may be said to apply to Macaura, the manufacturers of the Vitalator, and to many other proponents of irregular therapies.[24]

We should also accept that it is unlikely in any period that contemporary medical accounts, whether conventional or unorthodox, were the only narratives of tuberculosis that lay people would have encountered. And even those narratives will themselves have been affected by non-medical ways of thinking about the disease. With fifty-three thousand deaths in Britain from tuberculosis in 1871 and twenty-three thousand even in 1947,[25] many people had relatives and associates who had suffered from the disease. People living in fear of the disease in the 1930s often had relatives in their grandparents' generation who had been treated under understandings of disease causation and processes that antedated germ theory. There is no compelling reason to believe that the laity would have had any more "up-to-date" beliefs about tuberculosis than about history, for example, where old ideas about the catastrophe of industrialisation, for instance, dominated the popular view of the industrial revolution through long periods in which university academics promoted much more melioristic accounts of the period.[26] Most striking of all is that belief in the heritability of tuberculosis persisted well beyond the Second World War. Fifty-five percent of survey respondents from three London boroughs in 1950 considered tuberculosis to be hereditary,[27] despite nearly sixty years of concerted health education from the National Association for the Prevention of Tuberculosis (NAPT) asserting the disease to be infectious, and not inherited.[28] Although scholars have described changes in medicine's approach to tubercular patients, it would be unwise to assume that these changes expunged older lay stories. Beliefs about heritability sat alongside stories of taint, as neighbourhoods campaigned against the siting of sanatoria in their vicinity and refused to employ cured consumptives. And, whatever the mixed view of causation, to become a consumptive carried enormous stigma in the first half of the twentieth century that set its sufferers apart, often spatially, by their dependence – even after cure – on the sanatorium.[29]

Culture in general was shot through with tuberculosis stories. It is a commonplace that the history of the novel is studded with tubercular characters, sometimes created by tubercular authors. We have only to call to mind Tristram Shandy and Laurence Sterne, the Brontës, Hans Castorp, and Thomas Mann.[30] This territory, incidentally mapped out by H.D. Chalke, is ripe for richer and more extensive exploration to chart its contours. We may imagine Roy Porter's lusty exploration of *Tristram Shandy,* combined with Jonathan Rose's forensic approach to the reading habits of working class autodidacts, as a means to navigate the literary influences on the storied subjectivity of those imagining tuberculosis as sufferers or as onlookers.[31] But that is a larger task than this chapter can undertake.

Beyond this, the disease had a profound metaphorical presence in culture more generally, as Susan Sontag showed in *Illness as Metaphor*. The metaphorical associations of consumption, which she decried, continued to be available as narrative components in individuals' "period storybooks": that tuberculosis was associated with Romantic poets, musicians, and artists; that the disease conveyed a superior sensibility; that looking tubercular – "pale and interesting" – became a mark of distinction. All these components continued to be reinforced by rereading and retelling in new media.[32]

TUBERCULOSIS STORIES IN THE MAINSTREAM CINEMA

One significant source of tuberculosis narratives in this period was the cinema, which, in Britain, eighteen million people per week attended in the mid-thirties.[33] From the exhaustive subject index of *The American Film Institute Catalog* it is possible to describe in outline the ways in which tuberculosis was represented in American films, which dominated the cinematic fare of British audiences from within two decades of cinema's invention in 1895. It lists under "tuberculosis" one film before 1910; twenty-nine between 1911 and 1920; seven between 1921 and 1930; fourteen between 1931 and 1940; and nine between 1941 and 1950.[34] Several stories feature strongly, inflected by means of different narratives. For example, there was an association between Irish ethnicity, slum-dwelling, criminal activity, and tuberculosis – as in *Let Them Live* (1937), in which the hero, Dr Paul Martin, saves the life of a child whose father had tried to gas his tenement-dwelling family, fearing a prolonged tuberculosis-induced death for them.[35] Some films narratives turned on the herdity of tuberculosis – in *The Nth Commandment* (1923), for example, the illegitimacy of a child is revealed by his having the disease, as his real father had before him. Other films featured irregular tuberculosis therapies, for example, King Vidor's *The Citadel* (1938). The climax of the film is marked by the decision of its hero, Andrew Manson, to send a patient to an unlicensed American tuberculosis expert, thereby risking being struck off the medical register.

In some films, such as *Of Human Bondage* (1934), moral decline and tuberculosis are linked – here "Mops" Collins, a woman of loose morals played by Bette Davis, gets tuberculosis and dies. In others, the presence of a tubercular character conveniently presents a plot point; so in John Ford's *The Plough and the Stars* (1937) the hero evades arrest for his part in the 1916 Dublin uprising against British rule by hiding his rifle in the coffin of a character who has recently died of the disease.[36] The British film industry also produced titles with strong tuberculosis themes, some very popular, including *Alfie* (directed by Lewis Gilbert, 1965; screenplay by Bill Naughton), and some less popular and therefore less influential in confirming or disrupting lay narratives, including *Twice Round the Daffodils* (directed by Gerald Thomas, 1962), described as a "romantic comedy about a group of nurse-chasing patients at a tuberculosis sanatorium."[37]

The point here is not so much that such incidental details determined lay beliefs as that they joined the "period storybook" of tuberculosis. Some of these details may have resonated with majority stories, for example that tuberculosis was associated with poverty; others might have reinforced common prejudice that particular nationalities, especially immigrants, were disease vectors. Beliefs in disease as retribution for wrongdoing may have rendered credible unfounded associations between tuberculosis and crime or depraved sexual morality. In other words, any one of these narratives might have spun threads in the web of stories about tuberculosis that any member of the laity carried in their heads.

PART TWO: LAY NARRATIVES AND TUBERCULOSIS HEALTH EDUCATION FILMS

The films so far described only incidentally contained tuberculosis narratives. I proposed above that when health educators present audiences with disease narratives, they enter an already narrated space in peoples' lives. Accordingly, I now want to change mode and turn to health education films, ones that specifically sought to alter audiences' views of tuberculosis. But first it is necessary to consider health education more generally in the light of the narrative approach I have been discussing. Health education in this context may be seen as the attempt to replace lay narratives of disease with medical ones. Health education – or "propaganda" as it was often called – was a child of the third historical phase of public health activity. The first phase was the environmental sanitation of Chadwick; the second saw the application of bacteriology through isolation, disinfection, and similar measures. The third era, of personal hygiene, which stretched from the early twentieth century, sought to recruit individual citizens to the prevention of disease by educating them about patterns of behaviour likely to cause disease.[38] Enthusiasts for health education adopted a wide variety of media including posters, leaflets, lectures, and the dominant popular medium of the day, films.[39]

All health education in the period under discussion – and arguably up to the present – rested on hierarchies of communication, both between government and people and between the knowledgeable and the ignorant. In the long-lasting model originally promoted in the mid-1920s by George Newman, first chief medical officer, expert proponents independent of the Ministry of Health were made responsible for undertaking health education.[40] In Newman's view this approach was necessary if the state was to avoid overstepping its mandate. As he put it, "governmental action is the outcome of public opinion, and this in turn is formed by the more educated section of the people and by individual exponents," which included voluntary health associations and filmmakers.[41] This approach rested on what has since become known in studies of the public understanding of science as the "deficit model," within which popularisation is seen as providing scientific facts to fill the empty vessels of the lay mind.[42]

In Newman's version, whilst popularisation of medical knowledge was given a democratic inflection, health education was a matter of providing factual truths that were expected to motivate the public to rational action. But an account, such as this essay proposes, that seeks to gain access to the experience of the public has to be not one that looks from the top of the communication hierarchy towards the public but one that looks from the point of view of the audience. Such an account is the model of cultural consumption proposed by the French writer Michel de Certeau. This model can be applied to discuss how individuals consume information such as health education. Speaking of perceptions of the types of elite producers of information (we may include health education), de Certeau states: "the elite ... always assumes that the public is moulded by the products imposed on it. To assume that is to misunderstand the act of 'consumption.' This misunderstanding assumes that 'assimilating' necessarily means 'becoming similar to' what one absorbs, and not 'making something similar' to what one is, making it one's own, appropriating or reappropriating it."[43] De Certeau proposes that cultural consumption is active and that consumers pick and choose – accept and reject – from cultural products that are designed to be absorbed whole. This analysis is congruent with the narrative approach discussed in this paper, in the sense that fragments of stories may well be assimilated into existing narrative patterns, while whole narratives – if they do not tally – may be rejected out of hand.

Eighteen tuberculosis health education films were in distribution in Britain until the Second World War, under the auspices of the National Association for the Prevention of Tuberculosis (NAPT), which was fulfilling its role as part of Newman's "more educated section of the people."[44] It goes without saying that these films articulated dominant medical views of the disease. Some, such as *The Production of Tuberculin-Tested Milk* (1935), showed precautions against the disease; others, including *Air and Sun* (1921), showed the therapeutic regime followed in Swiss alpine resorts. Others told the stories of people with tuberculosis.[45]

The distinction between showing and telling that we encountered above in relation to written accounts also applies to films. The address of fictional films – such as those discussed in the previous section – works by showing (that is, it is mimetic), in that it creates a fictional world in which the content is carried by the actions and speech of characters within the plot. Members of the audience are expected to identify with the characters in the film. The events of the film are "overheard," as it were, from conversations between characters. Commonly there is no narrator outside the characters in the film, and therefore the audience is not addressed directly by anyone in the film, on-screen or off.[46] The diegetic, or telling, mode of address, on the other hand, is typically found in non-fiction films. In this case, commentators most often communicate the "message" of the film directly to the audience. The same distinctions also applied to silent films, the dominant form in the cinema for its first thirty years, although here the mimetic, storied, approach was most often taken, with acting styles and captions conveying the characters' subjectivity.

As with the majority of voluntary health associations, the NAPT often chose to present their health education through mimetic fictional stories using moral narratives (often featuring sequences of innocence, transgression, punishment, and atonement). These included the earliest film, *The Story of John M'Neill*, made at the

Royal Victoria Hospital in Edinburgh by the medical doctor Halliday Sutherland in 1911 and shown by the NAPT from 1924 and throughout the 1930s. Here, a narrative form was employed to convey the film's intended message, representing both the infectiveness of the disease and sanatorium life. The opening of the film has the slum-dwelling M'Neill family infected by the mother, who is shown unwarily sharing eating utensils and spitting. After the daughter, suffering early tuberculosis, attends a dispensary, a nurse visits the home and cleans and advises; a doctor examines the whole family and arranges for their treatment. Most of the second reel is taken up with details of John M'Neill's regimen in the sanatorium. He is returned cured to his family and then gains work on a farm through the local care committee and takes his children with him. A caption board reads, "in their new home the M'Neills will carry on the lesson they have been taught whilst under treatment – that fresh air, sunshine, cleanliness, and regular habits and suitable food, prevent the disease and that quack remedies are no good."[47] This silent film presents the narratives of several characters that audience members might identify with: the ignorant and culpable mother, the responsible daughter, and John M'Neill himself, whose personal narrative is the main vehicle for illustrating the process of cure.

Considerable numbers of people were shown these NAPT-distributed films. Like several other voluntary health associations, the NAPT owned specialised transport devoted to showing films across the country, in their case from 1928 to 1946. The driver visited wide geographical areas to show the films. For example, between January and September 1944 in the South East and the Midlands, he showed films to audiences of 31,300 children and 19,100 adults.[48] *Stand Up and Breathe* (1935), a departure for the association in terms of its approach (positive health, rather than their more usual fare of sanatorium life), its production values (on this occasion the association employed a commercial company, British Utility Films, rather than making the film itself), and its cinema showings, enjoyed audiences of 134,000 in its first two months.[49]

DEFEAT TUBERCULOSIS

Having looked at the presence of tuberculosis narratives within culture and at tuberculosis health education films in general, it remains for us to consider a particular storied tuberculosis film. For this study, I take the example of *Defeat Tuberculosis*, made for the

British Ministry of Health and released in 1943. Several different groups had put forward suggestions for films on tuberculosis from October 1941 onwards.[50] Finally, in March 1942, the Ministries of Health and Information (MOH, MOI) agreed to the production of *Defeat Tuberculosis* as a non-theatrical film (that is, one made to be shown in places other than cinemas, including town halls, factories, schools, and church halls, by medical officers of health or in MOI programs).[51] This approach was the result of the new wartime system of producing health education films through the MOI, rather than delegating responsibility to voluntary health associations.

The MOI approached the production company Seven-League on behalf of the MOH in April 1942 to prepare a treatment for the film. The company was commissioned to prepare a shooting script at the end of June, and it was ready a month later.[52] The director was Hans Nieter, proprietor of the company, trading from the same address as Paul Rotha, the well-established documentarist, who acted as its producer.[53] Diagrams were supplied by Otto Neurath of the ISOTYPE Institute, who worked with Rotha on at least a dozen films commenced during the war.[54] Rotha had already produced films on diphtheria immunisation and blood transfusion for the Ministry of Health. His company was a likely choice as it specialised in "films about progress in the fields of education, health, medicine, housing and the social sciences".[55] But the choice of film-makers was also ideologically and aesthetically congenial to Ministry of Health officials who had favoured documentary over other genres for *Health for the Nation*, a prestige film on the work of the ministry in 1938–39.[56]

The July 1942 shooting script for the film starts with a short historical vignette "a hundred years before" with a "hopeless case" of consumption. The main part of the script represents contemporary tuberculosis policy by telling the literal narrative of two sisters, Betty (who works in a factory's office) and Joan (who works on its shop floor). Most of the film was to be conveyed by mimetic synchronised dialogue between the sisters, their GP, and doctors at the tuberculosis dispensary and sanatorium.[57] For the audience, especially young women in industrial occupations, the film was intended to work by way of identification with the story of Joan and Betty, in order to propose how they, as potential tuberculosis sufferers, should act. We may note that although there had been a minor strand of using fictional, mimetic scenarios in documentary since *Pett and Pott* (Alberto Cavalcanti, for the GPO Film Unit, 1934), *Defeat Tuberculosis* was one of the first *documentary* health education films to set out to use a fictional scenario.

In the narrative, Betty's work has been suffering, so her employer suggests she visit the doctor, and her sister agrees to go with her. The GP, Dr Jeakins, prescribes a tonic for anaemia and notes that Joan is coughing. He says, "I don't want either of you to have the slightest doubt in your mind ... so I'm going to send you round to the tuberculosis dispensary ... both of you ... for an x-ray. It's quite simple and only takes a couple of minutes." In the voice of the doctor, the script directly addresses the question of heredity: "just because your mother died of tuberculosis there's no reason to think that you must have it. IT IS NOT HEREDITARY. But ... you can catch it". In this version Jeakins was to explain mass radiography. At the dispensary, Dr Walker clears Betty but detects signs of tuberculosis on Joan's lung. This narrative detour – that it's Joan (the machine operator) who has tuberculosis and not the secretary, Betty – is a feature of the disruptions to story sequence that Cobley describes as "typical of all but the most rudimentary narratives." In direct speech, Dr Walker explains that sanatorium stays are covered by health insurance or local authority doles and that she will receive artificial pneumothorax treatment. The brief section of narration about isolation is followed by dialogue between the sisters and Dr Bryan, the sanatorium doctor. Finally, after an Isotype sequence (a system of pictograms) on the dangers of delay, with a change to a close-up on Dr Bryan, his mode of address changes to the second person: "You see to-day we doctors know how to detect, fight and cure tuberculosis, but we can do nothing unless *you* all help" (my emphasis).

Then, in a deliberately jarring change in mode of address that was presumably intended to mark the transition from showing (mimetic) to telling (diegetic), the camera moves to show that Dr Bryan is speaking from a cinema screen. He proceeds to address people in the audience: "Tuberculosis can attack any of you, wherever you come from, or whoever you are ... it may attack you Mrs Jones – or you Mr Smith ... and you too Mary Brown ... you too, George." He continues to explain that neither poverty nor bad housing nor weakened health nor working and living conditions can cause tuberculosis without "the germ." He invokes joint, citizenly action: "It's *our* business to see that we stamp out tuberculosis

... we must stamp out slums, and poverty, and overcrowding – and we must see to it ... that never again will we allow conditions that encourage the spread of infection ... that's one of our peace aims." Dr Bryan then moves into the imperative: "Get as much fresh air as you can. Use your handkerchief if you want to cough, sneeze or spit, and so prevent possible infection." The film ends with him voicing a caption: "If you have a cough that lasts for several weeks go and tell a doctor. DO NOT PUT IT OFF. Probably there is nothing wrong – but if there is, you may endanger others near and dear to you."

Production was commissioned in August 1942, and the film was said to be complete in early October.[58] But *Defeat Tuberculosis* was not released for another eleven months, in September 1943.[59] Evidence to explain the delay is patchy, and it may well have been the result of rapidly evolving tuberculosis policy, but between the shooting script and the release, the film underwent several significant alterations.[60] The most striking was in its narrative approach: the released version replaced most of the direct mimetic speech sequences between the sisters, and even those in the mouths of the doctors, with an authoritative male voice-over that describes the speech and meaning of the actions on screen. Only the sequences before the sisters go to the GP retain the synchronised dialogue. A general rule in film production is that where economy of production is a factor, as here, it is synchronised mimetic dialogue sequences that are likely to be lost. The cheapest solution available to film producers where a film has to be altered is to use film sequences already shot and to record a new soundtrack – to record new scenes with synchronised sound involves much greater expense and complexity in re-recruiting actors, for example.

Whatever the cause, the result was that the showing (mimetic) mode had been almost entirely replaced with the telling (diegetic) mode. I suggest that in the terms of the analysis presented in this chapter this change is significant. Audience members were being asked to identify with a narrative subjectivity of citizenly good behaviour, and yet the supposed vehicle of audience identification, mimetic dialogue, had been almost entirely excised. The story of Joan and Betty – designed to correct audience misapprehensions – had survived, but it had lost the supposedly more effective mimetic mode of address to members of the audience. Certainly the shock value of the change to the diegetic mode at the film's conclusion had been very diminished by these changes.

Tens of thousands of people saw *Defeat Tuberculosis* from autumn 1943 onwards; so valuable was it seen to be that a new version was produced in 1950.[61] The data on the reception of this particular film are, however, less than sparse. The effectiveness of health education in changing lay beliefs – whether through individual films or whole campaigns – was scarcely evaluated at all in this period. But in the small number of studies that began to be undertaken in the 1940s, it is clear that although hundreds of thousands may have seen particular films, they do not appear to have registered particularly strongly in respondents' minds. For example, the Wartime Social Survey's study of the 1941–42 Autumn Health Campaign revealed that only 18 percent could remember seeing the health films that were widely shown as parts of ordinary cinema programs.[62] Such evidence, coupled with the persistence of lay belief in heritability, justifies a sceptical assumption about the success enjoyed by tuberculosis health education.

We have no specific evidence of how audience members accommodated the narrative of *Defeat Tuberculosis* to their own stories about the disease.[63] It is characteristic of the period that records of showings of health education films report only numbers attending. So far no specific evidence of precise numbers attending showings has come to light. We may, however, in the spirit of the analysis presented in the first part of this essay, quizzically consider elements of the narrative. Is it likely that the 55 percent whose tuberculosis narratives held the disease to be hereditary would have changed their minds on the strength of the final commentary asserting, "Now the real reason why Betty doesn't want to go to the doctor is because two years ago her mother died of tuberculosis. The doctor tells her you can't inherit tuberculosis; it's not hereditary"? Equally, being told not to be afraid of going to the doctor, or of having a chest x-ray, may well not have shifted one of the dominant stories of the era, namely that having tuberculosis and going to a sanatorium was life-changingly disruptive. Other narrative strands that we have discussed could also have crowded in to reduce the impact of the film: the narratives that it's not people like me, but those supposedly deserving punishment for moral lapses, such as Irish hoodlums or those that break the law or "pale and interesting" artists or Bette

Davis acting the floozy, that get the disease. We don't need to believe that cultural narratives necessarily *cancel* health education messages. But we should acknowledge that a complex narrative interaction occurs when new stories are imposed on already narrated areas of peoples' lives.

CONCLUSIONS

This chapter has shown that ideas of tuberculosis in the past were storied. In the second part I have set out to problematise how storied forms encapsulated in health education films may have been received by the public, given the wide range of tuberculosis narratives available to them. In the section "Defeat Tuberculosis" I have shown that the forms of health education narratives presented to the public are as subject to contingency as any other aspect of the public health and medical practices of which they are a part.

It remains to consider how this narrative approach relates to more empirical attempts at grasping lay subjectivity about disease. As I have shown, many tuberculosis stories and narratives existed within the culture of the era before effective chemotherapeutics. But compared with the kinds of written sources that historians are accustomed to use, the stories that *individuals* told have by nature been recorded less often and are therefore more diffusely scattered through the historical record. As historians we must recognise that the written record has been made for specific reasons – first, to ensure follow-up of patients, perhaps, and maybe later to tell the "biography" of a sanatorium, or to preserve the public relations correspondence of a ministry, first for reference, then for historical record. There is no ready empirical and direct access to the narratives lay people told themselves in the past, except by highly diligent archival research, like that undertaken about patients by Rothman in particular. If we were to seek access to such narratives through oral history, we would necessarily acquire narratives convenient to the time of telling, rather than to the time described.

However, just as David Lodge has suggested in *Consciousness and the Novel* that the free indirect mode in literature can be seen to provide special access to the consciousness of fictional characters and therefore authors, so this mode may also prove the most valuable evidence of consciousness *about disease*. First-person narratives may shine through by means of the free indirect mode within formal histories, as we saw with the Frimley example, or even, occasionally, in the records of bureaucracies. I propose that, whilst the search for empirical verification might well be valuable, the narrative approach I have proposed can comfortably sit alongside established social-historical approaches, offering a further corrective to the top-down over-medicalised, bureaucracy-centred views of diseases within culture that both written archives and the histories that rest on them tend to reinforce.

NOTES

1 F.B. Smith, *The Retreat of Tuberculosis, 1850–1950* (London: Croom Helm 1988); J. Harley Williams, *Requiem for a Great Killer* (London: Health Horizon 1973); Thomas McKeown, *The Role of Medicine: Dream, Mirage or Nemesis?* (London: Nuffield Provincial Hospitals Trust 1976).

2 Linda Bryder, *Below the Magic Mountain: A Social History of Tuberculosis in Twentieth-Century Britain* (Oxford: OUP 1988); Smith, *Retreat*; Sheila M. Rothman, *Living in the Shadow of Death: Tuberculosis and the Social Experience of Illness in America* (New York: Basic Books 1994); Katherine Ott, *Fevered Lives: Tuberculosis in American Culture since 1870* (Cambridge, MA: Harvard University Press 1996).

3 Susan Sontag, *Illness as Metaphor and Aids and Its Metaphors* (London: Penguin Books 1991), 3.

4 See David Armstrong, "The Doctor-Patient Relationship: 1930–1980," in Peter Wright and Andrew Treacher (eds.), *The Problem of Medical Knowledge: Examining the Social Construction of Medicine* (Edinburgh: Edinburgh University Press 1982), 109–22; Anne Digby, *Making a Medical Living: Doctors and Patients in the English Market for Medicine, 1720–1911* (Cambridge: Cambridge University Press 1994); Lilian R. Furst, *Between Doctors and Patients: The Changing Balance of Power* (Charlottesville: University Press of Virginia 1998); Roy Porter (ed.), *Patients and Practitioners: Lay Perceptions of Medicine in Pre-Industrial Society* (Cambridge: Cambridge University Press 1985).

5 Howard Brody, *Stories of Sickness* (Oxford: Oxford University Press 2003); Trisha Greenhalgh and Brian Hurwitz (eds.), *Narrative Based Medicine: Dialogue and Discourse in Clinical Practice* (London: BMJ Books 1998), 5.

6 David Armstrong, *Political Anatomy of the Body* (Cambridge: Cambridge University Press 1983), 80–2; Michael Balint, "The Doctor, His Patient, and the Illness," *The Lancet* (1955): 683–8.

7 Mildred Blaxter, *Health and Lifestyles* (London: Routledge 1990); Clive Seale, Stephen Pattison, and Basiro Davey, *Medical Knowledge: Doubt and Certainty* (Buckingham: Open University Press 2001), 24–5; Lola Romanucci-Ross, "The Hierarchy of Resort in Curative Practices: The Admiralty Islands, Melanesia," *Journal of Health and Social Behaviour* 10 (1969), 201–9.

8 See Tim Boon, *Films and the Contestation of Public Health in Interwar Britain* (London, University of London, unpublished PhD thesis), passim; Mariel Grant, *Propaganda and the Role of the State in Inter-War Britain* (Oxford: Oxford University Press 1994); Bridget A. Towers, "Health Education Policy, 1916–1926: Venereal Disease and the Prophylaxis Dilemma," *Medical History* 24 (1980): 70–87.

9 See below. I covered some of this in my unpublished paper "With Pig and Parachute in Search of the Audience for Interwar Health Education Films," presented to the conference Health Promotion in Historical and Contemporary Context," University of East Anglia, Norwich, 27 April 2001.

10 Paul Ricoeur, *Time and Narrative*, 3 vols., translated by K. McLaughlin and D. Pellauer (Chicago: University of Chicago Press 1990), 52; quoted in Brody, *Stories*, 24.

11 Paul Cobley, *Narrative* (London: Routledge 2001), 5–6.

12 Ibid., 2.

13 David Lodge, *Consciousness and the Novel* (London: Secker & Warburg 2002), 37.

14 For the general point about clinical narratives, see Stuart Hogarth and Lara Marks, "The Golden Narrative in British Medicine," in Greenhalgh and Hurwitz, *Narrative Based Medicine*, 140–8.

15 Armand Trousseau, *Lectures on Clinical Medicine*, translated by John Rose Cormack (from 1868 ed.) (London: New Sydenham Society 1870), vol. 3, 155–7. Armand Trousseau (1801–67) was professor of clinical medicine in the Faculty of Medicine, Paris.

16 H.D. Chalke, "The Impact of Tuberculosis on History, Literature and Art," *Medical History* 6 (1962): 301–18, 309.

17 Nicholas Jewson, "Disappearance of the Sick-Man from Medical Cosmologies, 1770–1870," *Sociology* 10 (1976): 225–44.

18 John R. Bignall, *Frimley: The Biography of a Sanatorium* (London: National Heart and Chest Hospital 1979), 68.

19 Galen Strawson, review of Jerome Bruner, "Making Stories: Law, Literature, Life," *Guardian Review*, 10 January 2004, 15.

20 Michael Baxandall, *Painting and Experience in Fifteenth Century Italy: A Primer in the Social History of Pictorial Style* (Oxford: OUP, 1988).

21 J.G. Macaura, *The Macaura Blood Circulator: Instructions & Useful Hints* (London: Macaura Institute, c.1920), Science Museum Registry, technical file A602776.

22 Leaflet supplied with Rogers Violet Ray Vitalator, c.1925, Science Museum Registry, technical file A602429.

23 J.B. Keswick, *The Herbal Family Guide*, rev. ed. (Wigton: J.B. Keswick & Co. 1935), 151.

24 Keswick, *Herbal Family Guide*, 201, 35. Smith, *Retreat,* devotes an extended section of his chapter "Responses" (56–91) to irregular therapies.

25 Smith, *Retreat*, 5.

26 Tim Boon, "History and Catastrophe: The Victorian Economy in British Film Documentary," in Michael Wolff and Miles Taylor (eds.), *The Victorians since 1901* (Manchester: Manchester University Press 2004), 107–20.

27 S.T. David, "Public Opinion concerning Tuberculosis," *Tubercle* 33 (1952): 78–90, 83–4, 89; discussed in Bryder, *Magic Mountain*, 221.

28 Bryder, *Magic Mountain*, 20–1.

29 Ibid.

30 Brody, *Stories*, 81–93.

31 Roy Porter, "'The Whole Secret of Health': Mind, Body and Medicine in Tristram Shandy," in John Christie and Sally Shuttleworth (eds.), *Nature Transfigured: Science and Literature, 1700–1900* (Manchester: Manchester University Press 1989), 61–84; Jonathan Rose, *The Intellectual Life of the British Working Class* (New Haven: Yale University Press 2001).

32 Sontag, *Illness as Metaphor*, chapter 4.

33 Simon Rowson, "A Statistical Survey of the Cinema Industry in Great Britain in 1934," *Journal of the Royal Statistical Society* 99 (1936).

34 American Film Institute and Kenneth W. Munden, *The American Film Institute Catalog of Motion Pictures Produced in the United States: Feature Films 1921–1930* (New York & London: R. R. Bowker Co. 1971–1999)[hereafter, AFC] 1911–20, 1029. Some films here, such as *The White Terror* (1915), were health education films made in association with the National Association for the Study and Prevention of Tuberculosis.

35 *AFC 1931–1940*, 1179–80.

36 *AFC 1931–1940*, 1671–2.

37 British Film Institute SIFT database; http://ftvdb.bfi.org.uk/sift/title/55601 (accessed 5 December 2006).

38 Paul Starr, *The Social Transformation of American Medicine* (New York: Basic Books 1982), 190–1.

39 Boon, *Contestation*, 10.

40 Ibid, 129–31.

41 George Newman, *Public Education in Health* (London: HMSO 1925), 17–18.

42 John M. Ziman, "Public Understanding of Science," *Science, Technology and Human Values* 16 (1991), 99–105.

43 Michel De Certeau, *The Practice of Everyday Life* (Berkeley: University of California Press 1984), 166.

44 Listed in appendix to Boon, *Contestation*, 317–18.

45 Health education films were often shown as adjuncts to lectures, and it is conceivable that this particular example accompanied lectures by Auguste Rollier in 1924. See *Report of the Bermondsey Medical Officer of Health*, 1924. For Rollier, see Bryder, *Magic Mountain*, 149–50.

46 Bill Nicholls, "Documentary Theory and Practice," *Screen* 17 (1976/77) 34–48, 38. See also Annette Kuhn, *Cinema, Censorship and Sexuality* (London: Routledge 1988), 49–74. Also David Pearson, "Speaking for the Common Man: Multi-voice Commentary in 'World of Plenty' and 'Land of Promise,'" in Paul Marris (ed.), *Paul Rotha* (London: BFI 1982), 64–85.

47 National Film and Television Archive, London, catalogue card; viewing of second reel; Bryder, *Magic Mountain*, 145.

48 Memorandum by J.H.Williams, 2 October 1944; report of film showings, 27 October, 1944; NAPT Propaganda Committee Minutes, Wellcome Archives, SA/NPT/A/3/5.

49 NAPT Propaganda Committee, 13 December 1935, Wellcome Archives, SA/NPT/A/3/3.

50 CCHE Films Sub-Committee, 31 October 1941, National Archives MH82/18.

51 March 1942 meeting, National Archives, MH78/234

52 Timings from memo by JKR, 25/9/51, National Archives, INF6/520 (The MOI record file for the film). Shooting script 3.2/266–268 preserved in Neurath, Isotype collection (MS109), University of Reading Archives. Final script in National Archives, INF6/1934. MH101/32, National Archives, for release date. See also Ministry of Health PR committee minutes, ninth meeting, 24 June 1942, National Archives, MH78/234.

53 This arrangement was followed with several Seven-League productions, including, for example, the film *Of One Blood* (1944).

54 For Rotha's collaborations with Neurath, see Tim Boon, *Films of Fact: A History of Science in Documentary Films and Television* (London: Wallflower Press 2008), 127–39.

55 Paul Rotha, "Documentary Films Yesterday and Today," press release appended to Paul Rotha to Julian Huxley, 11 February 1941, Julian Sorrell Huxley Papers, 1899–1980, Rice University, Houston, Texas.

56 Boon, "History and Catastrophe."

57 In this script, diegetic narration was limited to two short sequences: the historical prelude and the accompaniment to a sequence on the sanatorium ward and an ensuing ISOTYPE sequence showing the effect of isolation of tuberculosis carriers.

58 Harley Warner memorandum, 9 October 1942, attached to NAPT Council Minutes, 19 Oct 1942, Wellcome Archives, SA/NPT/A/2/1/9.

59 "Ministry of Health: New Tuberculosis Film Available," Ministry of Health War Diary, 23 September 1943, National Archives, MH101/32.

60 The shooting script encapsulated tuberculosis policy as it stood in mid–1942 and reflects the deliberations of the Standing Advisory Committee on Tuberculosis in Wartime, which, in February 1941, had been asked by Wilson Jameson, then chief medical officer, to "consider the examination, including mass radiography, of female industrial workers in the age group 15–24," like Joan. (Minutes of Standing Advisory Committee on Tuberculosis, 14 February 1941, MH55/1183; NAPT Council Minutes, 19 October 1942, SA/NPT/A/2/1/9; MH55/1183, passim.) We can see *Defeat Tuberculosis* as an incidental product of increasing centralisation of powers within the state during the Second World War and as a move away from the interwar mixed economy of private and public provision of health services, in which the ministry held an uneasy truce between two factions: those committed to private medicine – including voluntary associations undertaking health education – and the promoters of state medical services. One dynamic of centralisation affected control of health education: after the Blitz, in the crisis circumstances of the Second World War, health education was gradually, and increasingly firmly, "nationalised." The other dynamic of centralisation relates to a second shift in sources of expertise favoured by the ministry. When the rather technocratic Wilson Jameson commissioned a substantial report on tuberculosis in wartime in October 1941, he turned not to the Standing Committee, but to his old associates at the Medical Research Council (PRO MH

55/1141, Jameson to Mellanby, 29 October 1941). It is evident that members of the Standing Committee felt slighted (Minutes of Standing Advisory Committee on Tuberculosis, 5 December 1941, MH55/1183.). The resulting report came out in September 1942, just as *Defeat Tuberculosis* was being completed.

61 National Archives, INF6/1934.

62 Report for Ministry of Health on the Autumn Health Campaign, 1942, National Archives, MH101/31.

63 However, it is possible that the psychological literature could provide further generic leads, in works such as Melanie C. Green, Jeffrey J. Strange, and Timothy C. Brock (eds.), *Narrative Impact: Social and Cognitive Foundations* (Mahwah, NJ: Lawrence Erlbaum Associates 2002).

3

Targeting Patient Zero

DAVID S. BARNES

INTRODUCING PATIENT ZERO

On 16 October 1990, New Yorkers found Patient Zero's haggard, gaunt face looking out at them from their morning paper, his empty gaze staring wearily into the distance. As part of a series on the resurgence of tuberculosis in the city, the *New York Post* featured on its front page a homeless man who, the paper claimed, had been spreading the disease up and down Manhattan for eight months:

> Leo Maker, homeless and a junkie, roamed the city for eight months spreading tuberculosis. Coughing and highly contagious, he left a trail of tuberculosis germs from the Bronx to the Battery while sleeping in Grand Central, panhandling on the IRT [Interborough Rapid Transit subway] – even loading produce trucks in Chinatown.

The newspaper presented this heedless vagrant ("Leo Maker" was a pseudonym) not just as individually dangerous but also as representative of the "new tuberculosis," a plague that had seemingly come back from the dead. This time, the disease that had long been thought vanquished in the United States and other wealthy countries was even more insidious and more fearsome than before, spreading all but unnoticed in the very capitals of American biomedicine and impervious to the most sophisticated pharmaceutical weaponry available. In an urban environment, the danger was ubiquitous, and its inherent invisibility made the identification of "carriers" such as Leo Maker all the more important:

tuberculosis is so rampant among the homeless in this city that
doctors warn that everyone is at risk of being exposed. The risk
is greatest in crowded, enclosed areas – in the subways, on
buses, elevators, even in hospital emergency rooms ... The carriers are living, working and roaming everywhere in the city –
even working as cooks in restaurants.[1]

The threat of the deadly disease was effectively personified by
this one homeless "carrier." For a day at least, Patient Zero had
been found. Periodically throughout the 1990s, a similar drama
would play itself out in cities across the United States – but in medical journals rather than in tabloid newspapers. New laboratory
techniques gave scientific credibility to the age-old impulse to fix
blame for contagion. Responding to the spread of infectious disease by attempting to identify individual culprits was hardly a new
tendency, but I will argue in this essay that, aided in part by technological advances, it gained new appeal in the context of the
late-twentieth-century resurgence of tuberculosis.

The 1990 New York Post article was accompanied by screaming
tabloid headlines such as "Tuberculosis Timebomb" and a map of
Leo Maker's habitual journey of death and destruction: each step in
the mundane, if unsavory, daily existence of a homeless man in New
York City was in this instance freighted with portents of doom.

Leo Maker panhandled on the IRT subway line, in Grand Central
Terminal, and at the Port Authority Bus Terminal. After sleeping in
his favorite park at Madison Square, he would walk downtown to
Delancey Street, where he would clean car windshields for a few
dollars before heading up to Houston Street to buy heroin. Periodically he supplemented his income down in Chinatown loading and
unloading vegetable trucks. "You can always get day work in Chinatown unloading Chinese vegetables," he told the Post reporter. "I
was sick and coughing all the time, but sometimes you gotta force
yourself to work," he added.[2]

The newspaper's vivid and shocking revelation of Leo Maker's
germ-strewn wanderings could scarcely help but arouse strong feelings of fear and loathing among healthy and respectable New Yorkers. Moreover, and perhaps on an even more fundamental level, this
contagious junkie (depicted in two photographs, so that readers
could see what the menace looked like) evoked powerful white fears
of African Americans, the homeless population, and the dirty and

dangerous urban environment in general. Whether they were physically dangerous or not, men such as Leo Maker were seen as culturally dangerous: they lived lives utterly antithetical to the urbane, civilized ideal of stability, cleanliness, and sobriety. The fact that this man carried around with him a literal microbial contagion only reinforced the sense among respectable New Yorkers that any contact with his ilk was somehow contaminating in a more general sense. Indeed, the headline of an accompanying article says it all: "Homeless Contaminate Public Areas."[3]

Rather than a victim of poverty, social injustice, lack of education, or even of contagion from the person who transmitted tuberculosis to him, Leo Maker became, by virtue of the way the problem was framed, the Patient Zero of a potential or actual tuberculosis outbreak. (The fact that an essentially endemic, chronic disease could be depicted as occurring in discrete "outbreaks" or "epidemics" is itself a contingent historical phenomenon laden with theoretical and practical ramifications, as will be discussed below.)

"Patient Zero" is not a term often used by epidemiologists, who prefer more scientific terms such as "primary case" (the initial case that started an outbreak) or "index case" (the first case in an outbreak or group of cases to come to the attention of investigators). The ultimate goal is the same, however: find the starting point of an epidemic, and you hold the key to limiting its spread – and to preventing future epidemics. The proposition is not groundless, but neither is it self-evident; it needs to be examined carefully. At what cost do we focus our attention on identifying culprits, or "index cases"? Does this strategy help or hinder the effort to address the underlying, long-term causes of infectious disease?

If there were an "index case" in the outbreak of public references to "Patient Zero," it would surely be the 1987 book *And the Band Played On*, in which Randy Shilts identified a promiscuous gay French-Canadian flight attendant named Gaetan Dugas as the possible source of the AIDS epidemic in North America.[4] For a time in the anxious early years of the AIDS crisis, this individual – irresponsible and seemingly voracious in his deviance – served as a convenient and compelling focal point for the fears of those who somehow felt threatened, despite knowing themselves to be "normal." The identification of this index case served simultaneously to rationalize the epidemic by assigning blame for its spread and to

reinforce already strong stigmas and stereotypes regarding homo-
sexuality. Lessons have been learned from the hysteria and prejudice of the early AIDS epidemic, and the importance of the political
work that has been done in the wake of that experience should not
be underestimated. Nevertheless, the epidemiological investigation
of tuberculosis in the 1990s raises the prospect that well-intentioned efforts to combat the spread of infectious disease by identifying discrete outbreaks and putative "index cases" may unwittingly
encourage both public health officials and the general public to
travel further down the road that leads to unproductive scapegoating and gratuitous punishment.

There is a difference, of course, between gratutitous, sensational-
istic spotlighting of blameworthy individuals (such as Leo Maker)
and attempts to identify individuals infected with tuberculosis in
order to target medical interventions where they are most urgently
needed. However, it is important to recognize that the danger of the
former lurks inherently and constantly in the latter and that targeted prevention can become punitive rationalization quite subtly,
without any conscious decision being taken.

Taken literally, the very notion of a Patient Zero of tuberculosis is
absurd. The spread of a disease that has been endemic in many
parts of the world for centuries, and evidence of which has been
found in prehistoric skeletons, could not possibly be traced to a single individual, no matter how contagious or irresponsible. But the
suggestion that a sick person might even unwittingly have spread a
disease to a previously unaffected population is enough for that person to be viewed as (and treated as) a de facto Patient Zero. Against
the backdrop of the historical decline of tuberculosis in the industri-
alized world, almost any noticeable local increase could give rise to
alarm and suspicion.

PATIENT ZERO'S PEDIGREE

Attempts to track down and confine potential spreaders of contagion have a long history in infectious disease control. Indeed,
although widespread use of the name Patient Zero may have originated with Shilts's identification of Dugas, the role of Patient Zero
has been played by countless unfortunate disease victims throughout history. Versions of contagionist etiologies prevailed in various
societies for centuries before the bacteriological revolution. Con-

tagionism always implies chains of transmission, and from plague to syphilis to cholera, public health authorities have often attempted either during epidemics or in retrospect to identify human vectors who might explain the otherwise mysterious spread of a disease through a community. Even if nothing could be done to stop an outbreak, finding a common denominator among cases — especially if that common denominator was also a common scapegoat — could provide reassurance by way of rationalization.[5]

The impulse to find culprits responsible for spreading disease only intensified when germs came onto the etiological scene. Bacteriology brought a qualitatively new precision to the identification of index cases, and in the first decade of the twentieth century, an Irish immigrant cook named Mary Mallon personified the newly threatening spectre of germ spreader in the American press. Unlike most Patient Zeroes, "Typhoid Mary" enjoyed good health; like too many of them, she endured stigma and persecution in the name of public health. In a time of intense anxiety about waves of filthy immigrants washing over American cities, her ethnicity marked her as suspect from the beginning, just as Leo Maker fit the social profile of a disease spreader in an era marked by fear of the homeless and the African American urban underclass.[6] Science did not create the stigma that defined Mary Mallon in the eyes of the American public, but it did ratify it.

In the case of tuberculosis, some health officials in Europe and North America argued after Koch's identification of the tubercle bacillus that treating patients in poor law infirmaries, sanatoria, or other special facilities could limit the disease's spread by isolating consumptives from the general population, whether the actual medical treatments were effective or not.[7] However, until the mid-twentieth century, tuberculosis remained so common that the idea of tracing particular "outbreaks" to individual sources made no sense. The far-fetched began to seem reasonable – even urgent – when, on the heels of the long and gradual decline of tuberculosis, the availability of effective therapeutic drugs made the disease seem no longer a fact of life with which one simply had to come to terms. The prospect of achieving real control over tuberculosis by finding and treating cases (even by force, if necessary) fundamentally changed the standards by which preventive policies were judged.

In his book *Contagion and Confinement*, Barron Lerner showed how well-intentioned attempts to limit the spread of tuberculosis among the homeless population of Seattle veered inexorably toward incarceration and punishment based on behavioral transgressions rather than on strict health-related criteria.[8] In this case, as in so many other historical examples, a marginal population was constructed as not only deviant but also dangerous, thanks to the threat of contagion. Like Mary Mallon, who was first imprisoned in New York in 1907, uncooperative patients were condemned to incarceration less because of the actual harm they caused than because the stigmatized class to which they belonged amplified the alarm raised by their bacteriological status.[9]

Even if such extreme policies never became entirely routine, each proposed or actual implementation of coercive measures can only have lowered the threshold and bolstered the rationale for possible subsequent use. In Seattle at mid-century, repressive legal expedients devised in the context of a perceived health emergency acquired the status of guiding precedent and governed future interventions. Ad hoc policies ostensibly devised for special circumstances became standard operating procedure – no longer a last resort used to prevent contagion in extremis but an everyday tool used to achieve everyday disciplinary ends.[10] Lerner's analysis suggests that identification and incarceration of potential spreaders of contagion are not necessarily dangerous in and of themselves, but become ethically dubious and even counterproductive when control of the patient's body and conformity with behavioral norms overshadow the health and overall well-being of both the patient and the population as a whole.

In many nations, including the United States, the continued decline of tuberculosis to nearly negligible rates in the 1960s and 1970s displaced the questions of identification and incarceration of potentially contagious consumptives from the agenda of public health officials. Their alarm was therefore all the greater when the disease reared its ugly head again beginning in the 1980s. The resurgence of tuberculosis, the deadly tandem it formed with AIDS, and the appearance of antibiotic-resistant forms of the disease were experienced not only as the return of a terrifying spectre, but also as an affront to the technical mastery of biomedicine and its institutions.[11] Especially disturbing was the possibility raised by drug resistance: that existing prophylactic and therapeutic methods might be incapable of containing the disease. This was a qualitatively new tuberculosis, and it seemed to call for a new armamentarium of tuberculosis control. Although many factors were identified at the time as contributing to the disease's frightening comeback, there was one culprit in particular that came to be targeted by physicians and health officials as a clear and present danger and the root cause of multi-drug-resistant (MDR) tuberculosis: patient "noncompliance."[12] If the failure of recalcitrant patients to complete their treatment regimens was the cause of drug resistance, then it stood to reason that the only hope for rescue lay in overcoming this recalcitrance. As a result, tuberculosis control efforts (at least in the United States) came to be oriented around two axes: first, interrupting chains of transmission and, second, ensuring by any means necessary that treatment regimens were rigorously followed.

PATIENT ZERO'S FINGERPRINT

Each of these elements depended on timely and reliable identification. Beginning in the early 1990s, the application of new technologies to the study of disease outbreaks created an entirely new field of inquiry, baptized "molecular epidemiology," which promised to revolutionize the age-old practice of identifying actual or potential sources of contagion. The tools of genetic analysis could be used, molecular epidemiologists claimed, to precisely map the transmission of disease from person to person by identifying not just particular bacteria but particular strains of bacteria in patients. One of the first studies to chart the territory of this new domain appeared in the *New England Journal of Medicine* in January 1992. A team of researchers led by Phillip Hopewell and Charles Daley of San Francisco General Hospital and Peter Small of Stanford University analyzed a single "outbreak" of tuberculosis in a San Francisco residential facility for people infected with HIV. During the last half of 1990, two patients already being treated for tuberculosis had been admitted to the facility, and between December 1990 and April 1991, twelve new cases of the disease were diagnosed among the residents.[13]

The researchers isolated *Mycobacterium tuberculosis* from the sputum samples of each patient, and used restriction fragment-length polymorphism, or RFLP (one of the methods of "DNA fingerprinting"), to profile the isolates. The isolates from each patient were numbered according to the date of initial diagnosis. The RFLP

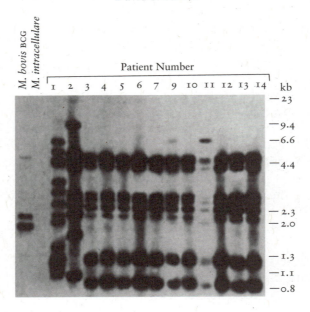

Figure 3.1
RFLPS of *M. bovis BCG*, *M. intracellulare*, and clinical mycobacterial isolates from residents of the HIV Congregate-Living Site

analysis revealed that Patients 1 and 2 (along with the random clinical isolates included as controls) had unique patterns, while 3 through 14 were essentially identical (figure 3.1). This meant that neither Patient 1 nor Patient 2 (who had entered the facility in 1990 already being treated for tuberculosis) was responsible for spreading the disease throughout the facility. Rather, it was Patient 3, who entered the facility in November 1990, who became the presumptive Patient Zero of this particular outbreak, having the first of the nearly identical strains to declare itself.[14]

The same group of researchers then went on to apply molecular epidemiological techniques to the overall incidence of tuberculosis in San Francisco. RFLP generated profiles of *M. tuberculosis* isolates from all patients reported to the San Francisco Department of Public Health's tuberculosis registry in 1991 and 1992. Of 473 patients in total, 191 grouped in what the authors called "clusters" – groups of two or more cases with essentially identical DNA profiles. The significance of the clustering phenomenon lay in the implication that a surprisingly large number of cases – every clustered case beyond the first in each cluster – represented recent infection or reinfection, rather than reactivation of latent infection. In this city-wide study, the RFLP data was supplemented by clinical records and by more traditional epidemiological techniques, including interviews and contact tracing. Intensive investigations were undertaken of the largest clusters and of the twenty clusters involving only two patients each.[15]

In some cases, the RFLP clusters confirmed groupings that were already known or could easily have been ascertained by old-fashioned epidemiology; some clusters, for example, involved individuals who lived or worked together or had close prolonged contact with one another. In others, however, the clusters didn't match common-sense groupings at all. This suggested to the researchers that *M. tuberculosis* could be transmitted relatively easily from person to person through brief, casual contact. The follow-up investigation of the largest cluster, involving thirty patients, is telling in this regard. This turned out to be the very same "outbreak" at the residential AIDS facility that the researchers had studied earlier – but it now appeared to have grown considerably, from a cluster of twelve to one of thirty patients with the identical strain. The city-wide analysis, in effect, turned up eighteen additional cases with the same fingerprint, none of which had any previously known connection with the AIDS facility. The study also gave this largest cluster a new Patient Zero:

> The apparent index patient in this cluster was a 38-year-old white man with AIDS who was receiving general assistance, was not compliant with anti-tuberculosis therapy, and had had positive sputum smears for approximately six months. Specific transmission links could be established among nine of the patients who were not associated with the residential facility; two named one another as contacts, three were on the same hospital ward, and four were in the same general medical clinic at a time when it was reasonable to assume that transmission had occurred. Although seven additional patients were homeless, homosexual, or substance abusers, they were not otherwise linked epidemiologically. Three patients had no discernible connection with any of the other patients.[16]

Arranging the cases chronologically by date of first tuberculosis diagnosis and supplementing the RFLP data with the interviews and

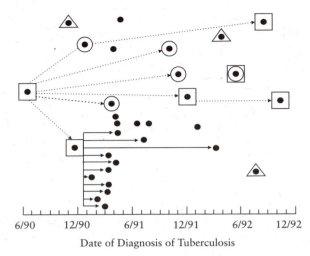

Figure 3.2
Transmission links identified between patients with isolates in the largest cluster. Each dot represents a patient. Solid lines indicate links between patients who were residents or employees of the same residential facility, dashed lines links between patients who were identified as contacts of other patients, and dotted lines links between patients who were in the same hospital ward, clinic, or homeless shelter at a time when transmission was likely to have occurred. Dots not connected to a line represent the seven patients for whom no specific epidemiologic connection could be discerned. Squares denote patients with cavitary tuberculosis and positive smears, circles patients with tuberculosis who had documented conversions of tuberculin skin tests within two years, and triangles patients for whom there was no discernible connection with any of the other patients.

inferences characteristic of conventional epidemiology, the investigators were able to plot with the precision and certainty of molecular biology the course of an outbreak from person to person within the city. The resulting diagram (figure 3.2) seems to herald a new era in the history of epidemiology. Like John Snow's map of the 1854 cholera epidemic around London's Golden Square, this graphical depiction possesses an eloquence and a sophistication that promised (or even equated with) mastery over disease.[17]

The next two largest clusters in the San Francisco RFLP analysis (consisting of twenty-three patients and fifteen patients, respectively) also originated, according to the researchers, with "noncompliant" patients: in one instance, an HIV-positive white transsexual prostitute and IV drug user and, in the other, an HIV-negative black alcoholic who frequented homeless shelters, detox centers, public clinics, hospitals, and other potential focal points for widespread

contagion.[18] The isolation of such clusters, combined with the identification of the index case, or Patient Zero, of each cluster, effectively shifted the terms of debate in tuberculosis control. Presented
in such a manner, the scientific data seemed to show that non-com-
pliant patients were infecting large numbers of people. How could
one look at this data and not feel that some kind of constraint or
coercion targeted against indiscriminate disseminators of bacteria
was called for? The decision to frame the epidemiological data in
terms of outbreaks, index cases, and lines of transmission makes
this all but a foregone conclusion. Identify past or present Patient
Zeroes, such studies seemed to hint, and we can not only prevent
them from doing further damage, but we can also take the first
steps toward pre-emptive action against potential future Patient
Zeroes. First identified, then closely monitored and treated – by
force if necessary – patients would be less likely to sow a "trail of
TB" in their wake.

A similar logic informs a 1995 study of a tuberculosis outbreak in
Minneapolis, Minnesota. In this case, however, the story began
rather than ended with the identification of Patient Zero. A forty-
eight-year-old homeless alcoholic showed up at a public hospital
one day in March 1992, unable to walk unassisted and suffering
from fever, chills, nausea, vomiting, diarrhea, cough, progressive
weakness, and severe weight loss. He reported that he spent most of
his days in a neighborhood bar, and slept either under a bridge, in
homeless shelters, or in the rooming house adjacent to the bar.[19]

Hospital, county, and University of Minnesota researchers undertook an extensive contact investigation (figure 3.3) centered on the
bar and rooming house. Four bartenders and ninety-three regular
customers were screened and tested to varying degrees. A total of
twenty cases of active tuberculosis eventually turned up in the
investigation, including six that were not part of the initial screening; all twenty showed RFLP patterns identical to that of the index
patient. Twenty- seven additional subjects in the investigation tested
positive for infection but remained asymptomatic. Although no
RFLP evidence existed for these individuals, the authors nevertheless concluded that they too had been infected by Patient Zero,
bringing his total to forty-one out of the ninety-seven contacts
screened, or 42 percent of contacts infected. The authors lamented
the fact that the index patient had never sought treatment and that
none of the bar's employees or customers had intervened at any

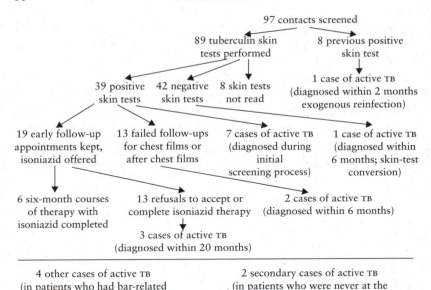

Figure 3.3
Flow-chart overview of the contact investigation and origin of the 20 active cases of tuberculosis that resulted from infection in the index patient.

stage, despite the proximity of both a public clinic and a public hospital to the bar. They noted that "[t]hough it would have been difficult, early intervention would probably have reduced the extent of the outbreak," and concluded that "[t]he spread of tuberculosis in a neighborhood bar can be a major public health problem."[20]

After the mid-1990s, the resurgence of tuberculosis gradually faded from public consciousness, and a slow but steady decline in new tuberculosis cases in the United States pushed the issue off the front pages of daily newspapers. Nevertheless, the hunt for Patient Zeroes in tuberculosis "outbreaks," "mini-epidemics," and "micro-epidemics" has continued, and the belief that effective tuberculosis control depends on identifying individual instances of transmission through molecular epidemiology has, if anything, solidified.[21] An outbreak in a "famous church gospel choir" in Newark, New Jersey, prompted another study combining DNA fingerprinting and conventional epidemiology. The tenor section was found to be at greatest risk of transmission, possibly because of its location during rehearsals. Once again, Patient Zero was identified as a homeless man; this one sang tenor in both the 8:00 A.M. and the 11:00 A.M. choirs and occasionally shared a ride to and from the church with a church elder and fellow tenor, who also became infected. The investigators concluded that old habits in research on the epidemiology of tuberculosis needed to change: "Conventional contact investigation must be supplemented by newer techniques, such as DNA fingerprinting, in identifying possible outbreak transmission ... Transmission need not only be in congregate settings among well-defined socioeconomic groups, but may occur unexpectedly in middle-class communities."[22] The gospel tenors' "miniepidemic" reinforces the (now familiar) lesson that homeless people are a threat to the health of the respectable middle class.

Even when DNA fingerprinting techniques have not been used to finger the culprit, specific instances of transmission have figured prominently in epidemiological studies of tuberculosis. When it was learned that a woman with an active and drug-resistant case of the disease had flown from Honolulu to Baltimore via Chicago to visit relatives, then returned by the same route a month later, the federal Centers for Disease Control (CDC) wondered how many fellow passengers she might have infected. A study was undertaken to contact and screen all of the passengers and crew members on each of the four legs of the patient's trip (Honolulu-Chicago, Chicago-Baltimore, Baltimore-Chicago, Chicago-Honolulu). Of 760 exposed contacts who could be reached, 29 had positive skin tests for tuberculosis infection. All but 6 of the 29 had also experienced either previous positive skin tests or known risk factors for infection other than their presence on one of the flights in question. The 6 passengers whose infection could not be accounted for by other factors had all flown on the final leg of the presumptive Patient Zero's journey: the flight from Chicago to Honolulu.[23]

When the CDC researchers consulted airline records and the plane's seating configuration (figure 3.4), they found that four of the six passengers believed to be infected on the fateful flight had been seated within two rows of Patient Zero. Further interviewing revealed that the other two infected passengers had frequently visited friends seated very near the sick woman and had used the lavatory located close to her seat. The CDC concluded that tuberculosis can be transmitted on long airplane flights and that the risk of infection is greatest among passengers seated in close proximity to a

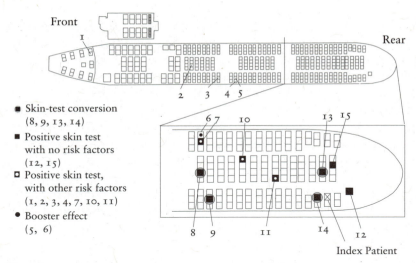

- ▣ Skin-test conversion
  (8, 9, 13, 14)
- ■ Positive skin test
  with no risk factors
  (12, 15)
- ▢ Positive skin test,
  with other risk factors
  (1, 2, 3, 4, 7, 10, 11)
- ● Booster effect
  (5, 6)

Index Patient

Figure 3.4
Diagram of the Boeing 747–100, with seat assignments of the passengers and flight crew on Flight 4 who had positive tuberculin skin tests. Contact 12 was a member of the flight crew.

passenger with active tuberculosis. The agency also suggested criteria for notifying passengers and crew after future instances of possible exposure to contagion: factors to be taken into account included the duration of the flight, the infectivity of the diagnosed disease, and the design of the aircraft. In certain circumstances, it was argued, notification of only those passengers and crew in the same cabin area as the patient might be adequate.[24]

Another study attempted to correlate tuberculosis infectivity with HIV status and intravenous drug use. Both household and non-household contacts of 248 patients with active tuberculosis (124 HIV-positive and 124 HIV-negative) were screened and tested for infection. It was determined that HIV-positive patients were twice as likely to transmit *M. tuberculosis* to contacts as were HIV-negative patients. Within the population of HIV-positive patients, IV drug users were almost four times as likely to infect contacts as were non-IV drug users. The authors of this study declared a "micro-epidemic" if a single index case was linked to two or more infections among contacts. Of the twelve microepidemics identified in the study, eight were caused by HIV-positive patients. According to the authors, the study "show[ed] the need for better preventive measures and tighter control of tuberculosis in HIV-infected patients, especially IV [drug users], through integrated programs that deal with the problematic issue of IV [drug use] with HIV and TB."[25]

Although not all of these Patient Zero-oriented studies relied on molecular epidemiology, all shared the conviction that tuberculosis control depends on the identification of potential germ spreaders. Meanwhile, other studies used the molecular genotyping of *M. tuberculosis* for purposes beyond identifying particular outbreaks, "microepidemics," or index cases. For example, in 1996 the CDC established the National Tuberculosis Genotyping and Surveillance Network, which consisted of seven "sentinel surveillance sites" throughout the United States. The network was designed to determine the extent to which typing distinct strains of the tubercle bacillus might "improv[e] ... TB prevention and control" by answering "specific epidemiologic questions regarding the natural history [and] transmission" of this microbe. When the time came to take stock of the project in a November 2002 special issue of the journal *Emerging Infectious Diseases*, researchers concluded that the experiment had shown significant promise. Several studies had shown correlations between particular ethnicities and certain tuberculosis genotypes; it was hypothesized that these correlations "may be useful in tracking the geographic origin and spread of [tuberculosis] strains of public health importance." The review concluded that the "widespread implementation" of DNA fingerprinting was "scientifically justified," and predicted that the technique "will be vital in the effort to eliminate TB." The authors left unspecified exactly how this "vital" role would be performed.[26]

SUPERSPREADERS AND OUTBREAK NARRATIVES

Public alarm in the United States over potential spreaders of tuberculosis such as Leo Maker and the Honolulu-bound airline passenger faded in intensity after the late 1990s, as the disease's incidence declined and other public health threats displaced it from the headlines. However, the epidemiological perspective that informed the earlier exposés of tuberculosis Patient Zeroes remains very much with us. When the world confronted the frighteningly unfamiliar disease that came to be known as sudden acute respiratory syndrome (SARS) in the spring of 2003, authorities applied reassuringly familiar patterns of thought to the challenge of containing the new contagion. During the short-lived pandemic, epidemiologists devised a new variant of the index case phenomenon: the "super-spreader" or "superinfector." Some patients seemed to display a unique capacity to infect large numbers of people, even through only brief, casual contact. Media accounts called the discovery of these "lethal virus vehicles" "[o]ne of the most frightening aspects of the SARS epidemic." "Virtually every major SARS outbreak is being traced to a single person or small number of patients," one news report claimed. The press also identified "the first 'super-spreader' to arrive in the Chinese capital," a twenty-seven-year-old businesswoman from Shanxi province who was promptly dubbed "Beijing's Patient Zero."[27]

Scientifically speaking, research into the characteristics of "super-spreaders" may be significant and original, though at first glance it bears a striking resemblance to the epidemiological tradition of Patient Zero identification. This work might even have immediate ramifications in public health policy, if the patients in question could somehow be identified and isolated in a timely manner. However, in the case of SARS, as with tuberculosis, the very notion of a "superspreader" further fuels the manifest impulse in time of perceived crisis toward prevention based on coercive or punitive measures. The suffering patient in need of care becomes, in effect, a dangerous suspect who must be contained. During the 2003 SARS pandemic, the Chinese government replaced its initial policy of denial and dissimulation with a draconian quarantine, with punishments of up to seven years in prison for violators – and the death penalty for anyone found intentionally spreading the disease.[28] In such a context, epidemiological techniques for tracking transmission cast an ominous shadow; one can only imagine what uses the Chinese authorities would make of some future test for identifying potential "superspreaders."

It would be unfair to tar all scientists and public health authorities with the same brush. Virologists and epidemiologists investigating the transmission of SARS bear no more direct responsibility for the harsh Chinese crackdown than the San Francisco molecular epidemiology researchers do for abuses of forced isolation or other coercive measures in tuberculosis control. Yet it is important to recognize the deep-rooted dynamic through which a particular epistemological orientation – one that sees the incidence of disease in terms of individual outbreaks and person-to-person transmission – inexorably calls forth policy responses aimed at preventing transmission at all costs, eclipsing other preventive strategies in the process.

Lest anybody conclude that tuberculosis Patient Zeroes lost their ability to frighten after the decline in tuberculosis incidence in the United States since the 1990s and the rise to prominence of SARS and other diseases, Atlanta lawyer Andrew Speaker can testify to the contrary. In May and June of 2007, reports that the thirty-one-year-old Speaker had flown to Europe for his wedding and honeymoon after being warned that he had drug-resistant tuberculosis ignited a firestorm of condemnation and hand-wringing. The heedless hedonist who had knowingly endangered hundreds of fellow airline passengers (not to mention others who crossed his path during his Aegean idyll) felt the full fury of the Patient Zero phenomenon. Cable TV programs and internet forums overheated with frenzied denunciations of "Tuberculosis Man," the "jackass" who had committed "attempted murder."[29] In the end, tests revealed that Speaker had infected nobody and did not in fact have an extensively drug-resistant strain of tuberculosis, as had been initially announced. Speaker's guilt, however, was undiminished. Like Mary Mallon and Gaetan Dugas before him, he had knowingly put others at risk; even worse, like Dugas, he had done so through his selfish pursuit of pleasure rather than through necessity or desperation.

The themes and tropes are now familiar. Patient Zero is a stock character in an oft-repeated drama of transgression, calamity, and (eventually) punishment. In a novel and important study, Priscilla Wald has recently called attention to the deep entrenchment of this paradigmatic story within American culture in the age of AIDS and other so-called emerging diseases. The classic "outbreak narrative," as Wald calls it, mobilizes threats, fears, hopes, villains, and heroes in the service of an important cultural purpose: reaffirming the bonds of social connection even while exposing their fragility and demonizing those who transgress their norms. Moreover, the narrative conventions of our familiar stories are of more than merely anecdotal or academic interest:

> Outbreak narratives ... have consequences ... They promote or mitigate the stigmatizing of individuals, groups, populations, locales (regional and global), behaviors, and lifestyles, and they change economies. They also influence how both scientists and

the lay public understand the nature and consequences of infection, how they imagine the threat, and why they react so fearfully to some disease outbreaks and not others at least as dangerous and pressing.[30]

When we look for index cases, or even when we conceptualize diseases in terms of discrete outbreaks constituted by individual acts of transmission, we cannot help but reproduce the conventions of the outbreak narrative. There may be very good reasons for framing disease in this way, but it is dangerous to do so without understanding the implications and potential ramifications.

CONCLUSION

Bane or boon? Judging the significance of molecular epidemiology and the search for index cases is not a simple matter. The potential drawbacks of these approaches must be weighed against the benefits they offer. For example, several of the initial studies discussed above that applied molecular epidemiology to tuberculosis outbreaks called attention to the surprising prevalence of recent infection or exogenous reinfection, rather than reactivation of latent infection, in the cases studied. This observation led them to recommend targeted surveillance of high-risk populations, along with prompt evaluation of contacts when individual cases arose. A greater incidence of cases due to reactivation, on the other hand, would instead have argued in favor of chemoprophylaxis for those with positive skin tests who might have been in danger of immunosuppression. This policy question might have remained an open one to this day in San Francisco or Minneapolis, for example, without this research, and scarce public health resources might have been inefficiently allocated. There may well be other potential benefits of this kind of knowledge that have yet to be demonstrated. Aside from anything else, the very idea that one could track through space and time the transmission of a particular genetic strain of a pathogenic bacterium is in and of itself somewhat breathtaking.

But at what what cost do such breakthroughs in epidemiological knowledge come? Does the unparalleled focus on the trees cause us to lose sight of the forest? An increasing emphasis on individual acts of transmission as contributing to specifically identifiable "outbreaks" runs the risk of obscuring the paramount etiological role of immunosuppression in tuberculosis. As control is equated more and more with the identification of potential spreaders, attention is diverted away from the disease's underlying causes. The factors that turn infection into disease – malnutrition, homelessness, alcoholism, drug abuse, and of course AIDS, among others – fade from visibility when transmission becomes everything. Each of the "outbreaks" mentioned in the studies discussed above involved homeless people, AIDS patients, and/or alcoholics. It would take a profound myopia to conclude that individual acts of tuberculosis transmission constitute the most salient public health problem in these circumstances or deserve to be the target of health authorities' energies. However, it is easier to suggest new ways to identify dangerous patients than to propose serious strategies to combat poverty, substance abuse, and other causes of immunosuppression.

The fledgling field of public health ethics has not had much to say about the impulse to target Patient Zero. One of its commonly enunciated principles, however, holds that coercive measures or the denial of individual rights are justifiable only when less restrictive preventive measures are not available and only when the fundamental causes of patient noncompliance are simultaneously addressed. Those scholars who have studied the real-life implementation of forced detention and other coercive anti-tuberculosis policies have found that they often fall short of this ethical standard. Even when motivated by the best of intentions and subjected to strict criteria, such measures have tended to slide past the bare minimum necessary for the protection of public health toward the punishment of noncompliance for its own sake.[31]

Wald's analysis of the outbreak narrative's internal dynamics, cultural resonance, and political ramifications points the way toward unlocking the conceptual straightjacket in which we find ourselves. If Gaetan Dugas had not existed, some have observed, he would have had to be invented. In fact, Wald argues, Dugas as Patient Zero *was* invented, "as a necessary component of the effort to write an HIV/AIDS outbreak narrative." Recognizing this fundamental truth and demonstrating its historical contingency, she shows, is the first step toward transcending it and building "more effective, just, and compassionate responses both to a changing world and to the problems of global health and human welfare."[32] Tracking "One Man's Trail of TB" is neither the only nor the optimal way to react to local increases in the incidence of tuberculosis.

In the final analysis, tuberculosis control strategies will prove themselves successful to the extent that they not only interrupt specific chains of transmission but generally improve the lives of the individuals and communities most at risk. When all is said and done, the homeless heroin addict Leo Maker is indeed an appropriate representative of the resurgence of tuberculosis and of the social breakdown that it signified. In tracking his hypothetical "trail of TB," we can't help wondering how many other cases this Patient Zero caused. But even as we reflect on that hypothetical danger, we would do well to ask who – or what – caused *his* tuberculosis.

NOTES

1 *New York Post*, 16 October 1990.
2 Ibid.
3 Ibid.
4 Randy Shilts, *And the Band Played On: Politics, People, and the AIDS Epidemic* (New York: St Martin's Press 1987). The original study implicating Dugas, which used the name "Patient 0" (possibly for the first time), appeared in 1984: M. Auerbach, W.W. Darrow, H.W. Jaffe, and J.W. Curran, "Cluster of Cases of the Acquired Immune Deficiency Syndrome: Patients Linked by Sexual Contact," *American Journal of Medicine* 76 (1984): 487–92.
5 See, for example, Terence Ranger and Paul Slack (eds.), *Epidemics and Ideas: Essays on the Historical Perception of Pestilence* (Cambridge: Cambridge University Press 1992); Ann G. Carmichael, "Contagion Theory and Contagion Practice in Fifteenth-Century Milan," *Renaissance Quarterly* 44 (1991): 213–56; and Guenter B. Risse, *Mending Bodies, Saving Souls* (New York: Oxford University Press 1999), 167–229. On the broader theme of rationalization, see David S. Jones, *Rationalizing Epidemics: Meanings and Uses of American Indian Mortality since 1600* (Cambridge: Harvard University Press 2004.
6 Judith Walzer Leavitt, *Typhoid Mary: Captive to the Public's Health* (Boston: Beacon Press 1996).
7 Leonard G. Wilson, "The Rise and Fall of Tuberculosis in Minnesota: The Role of Infection," *Bulletin of the History of Medicine* 66 (1992): 16–52, and "The Historical Decline of Tuberculosis in Europe and America: Its Causes and Significance," *Journal of the History of Medicine and Allied Sciences* 45 (1990): 366–96; Simon Szreter, "The Importance of

Social Intervention in Britain's Mortality Decline c.1850–1914: A Re-interpretation of the Role of Public Health," *Social History of Medicine* 1 (1988): 1–37.

8 Barron H. Lerner, *Contagion and Confinement: Controlling Tuberculosis along the Skid Road* (Baltimore: Johns Hopkins University Press 1998), 116–38.

9 Leavitt, *Typhoid Mary.*

10 Lerner, *Contagion and Confinement.*

11 Frank Ryan, *The Forgotten Plague: How the Battle against Tuberculosis Was Won – and Lost* (Boston: Little, Brown and Company 1992); Matthew Gandy and Alimuddin Zumla (eds.), *The Return of the White Plague: Global Poverty and the "New" Tuberculosis* (London: Verso 2003).

12 Paul Farmer et al., "Tuberculosis, Poverty, and 'Compliance': Lessons from Rural Haiti," *Seminars in Respiratory Infections* 6 (1991): 254–60.

13 Charles L. Daley et al., "An Outbreak of Tuberculosis with Accelerated Progression among Persons Infected with the Human Immunodeficiency Virus: An Analysis Using Restriction-Fragment-Length Polymorphisms," *New England Journal of Medicine* 326 (1992): 231–5.

14 Ibid.

15 Peter M. Small et al., "The Epidemiology of Tuberculosis in San Francisco: A Population-Based Study Using Conventional and Molecular Methods," *New England Journal of Medicine* 330 (1994): 1703–9.

16 Ibid.

17 Ibid. On Snow, his context, and his place in the history of epidemiology, see John Snow, *Snow on Cholera* (New York: Commonwealth Fund 1936), and "John Snow: A Historical Giant in Epidemiology," http://www.ph.ucla.edu/epi/snow.html.

18 Small et al., "Epidemiology of Tuberculosis."

19 Susan E. Kline et al., "Outbreak of Tuberculosis among Regular Patrons of a Neighborhood Bar," *New England Journal of Medicine* 333 (1975): 222–7.

20 Ibid.

21 For example, the number of articles with the subject term "pulmonary tuberculosis" and keywords "index case" in the Medline database of published medical literature began increasing above one per year in 1985 and has averaged over five per year since, peaking at ten in 1999. The first article with the subject term "pulmonary tuberculosis" and keywords "molecular epidemiology" appeared in 1993, and the number increased fairly steadily thereafter, peaking at nine in 2002.

22 Bonita T. Mangura et al., "*Mycobacterium tuberculosis* Miniepidemic in a Church Gospel Choir," *Chest* 113 (1998): 234–7.

23 Thomas A. Kenyon et al., "Transmission of Multidrug-Resistant *Mycobacterium Tuberculosis* during a Long Airplane Flight," *New England Journal of Medicine* 334 (1996): 933–8.

24 Ibid.

25 Joan A. Caylà et al., "The Influence of Intravenous Drug Use and HIV Infection in the Transmission of Tuberculosis," *AIDS* 10 (1996): 95–100.

26 Barbara A. Ellis et al., "Molecular Epidemiology of Tuberculosis in a Sentinel Surveillance Population," *Emerging Infectious Diseases* [serial online] 2002 Nov [29 *June 2004*], 8. Available from http://www.cdc.gov/ncidod/EID/vol8no11/02–0403.htm.

27 Shankar Vedantam, "A Single Patient Can Prove Lethal: Small Number Spread Disease Widely," *Washington Post*, 13 April 2003; Philip P. Pan, "A 'Superspreader' of SARS: How One Woman Touched Off Beijing Outbreak," *Washington Post*, 29 May 2003.

28 Philip P. Pan and John Pomfret, "China Threatens Death for Willful Spread of SARS," *Washington Post*, 16 May 2003.

29 These are just a few examples of the colorful language in which the Speaker case was discussed publicly. The *Denver Post*'s website attached the headline "Tuberculosis Man" to the discussion forum in response to a 30 May 2007 article about Speaker's travels and treatment: http://neighbors.denverpost.com/viewtopic.php?f=8&t=6016263. The 31 May 2007 entry of the blog "Granite Rock Sound" was entitled "A Jackass with Highly Drug Resistant TB or Andrew Speaker: Patient Zero": http://graniterocksound.blogspot.com/2007/05/jackass-with-highly-drug-resistant-tb.html. (A Google search on 5 August 2008 for the terms "Andrew Speaker" and "jackass" yielded 355 hits.) Many TV commentators, blogs, and discussion forums called for Speaker to be charged with attempted murder; see, for example, the transcript of the Cable News Network program CNN *Newsroom* that aired on 1 June 2007: http://transcripts.cnn.com/TRANSCRIPTS/0706/01/cnr.06.html.

30 Priscilla Wald, *Contagious: Cultures, Carriers, and the Outbreak Narrative* (Durham, NC: Duke University Press 2008), 3.

31 Barron H. Lerner, "Catching Patients: Tuberculosis and Detention in the 1990s," *Chest* 115 (1999): 236–41; R. Bayer and L. Dupuis, "Tuberculosis, Public Health, and Civil Liberties," *Annual Review of Public Health* 16 (1995): 307–26; Len Doyal, "Moral Problems in the Use of Coercion in Dealing with Nonadherence in the Diagnosis and Treatment of Tuberculosis," *Annals of the New York Academy of Sciences* 953 (2001): 208–15; Richard Coker, "Just Coercion? Detention of Nonadherent

Tuberculosis Patients," *Annals of the New York Academy of Sciences* 953 (2001): 216–23, and *From Chaos to Coercion: Detention and the Control of Tuberculosis* (New York: St Martin's Press 2000), 118.

32 Wald, *Contagious*, 3, 232, 254.

4

Beyond the Total Institution: Towards a Reinterpretation of the Tuberculosis Sanatorium

FLURIN CONDRAU

INTRODUCTION

When Erving Goffman published his seminal study *Asylums* in 1961, few would have anticipated its far-reaching impact on social theory and, somewhat later, the historiography of medical institutions.[1] Such institutions had previously been regarded as loci of care. But with Michel Foucault and Thomas Szasz, Goffman popularised the view that they ought to be studied as social institutions that shaped medical knowledge. Szasz coined the term *institutional pathology* to begin to understand what he called a misguided definition of (mental) illness. For him, institutions combined a general inability to usefully treat a mental illness with an explicit aim to educate and discipline defiant behaviour.[2] While much of this writing was initially confined to the anti-psychiatry movement of the 1960s, the new critique of modern medicine gave Goffman and the other authors an audience during the 1970s.

The most developed such analysis, the *nemesis of medicine*, by Ivan Illich, presented the shortfalls of medicine through a historical analysis of medicalization.[3] Much of his writing is strongly indebted to Marxist thought, which has shaped the modern view of the hospital as a health factory. But for the purpose of this chapter, Illich's study is most notable for its strong recurrence to history and historical thought to engage critically with the merits of modern medicine. Similarly, Foucault's analysis of the power of expert knowledge, undertaken very much as a historical sociology of science, has profoundly shaped the modern history of medical knowledge. Also, Thomas McKeown's analysis of the mortality decline has contrasted the promises of modern therapeutic medicine with its own historical record and emphasised the ineffectiveness of medicine over much of the eighteenth, nineteenth, and twentieth centuries.[4] Goffman's case, however, was different. His analysis of modern medical institutions was to a large extent driven by direct observation from working as a resident scientist in a large mental-health hospital, St Elizabeth's hospital in Washington, DC. This institution, with up to seven thousand inmates, the majority of Afro-American origin, clearly inspired his work on asylums.[5] Goffman crucially mirrored Szasz's assessment that much mental illness had no empirical or medical basis but largely existed to justify the medico-legal system. But where Szasz engaged with disease categories and questionable medical practice, Goffman focused on the institutions themselves and coined the term of a total institution as his starting point: "A Total Institution may be defined as a place of residence and work where a large number of like-situated individuals, cut off from the wider society for an appreciable period of time, together lead an enclosed, formally administered round of life."[6]

Goffman not only dismissed any medical function of such hospitals, asylums, and prisons, but he went on to declare that the single most important purpose of a total institution was the compulsory reconstruction of identity. This became really important for historians in the 1970s, when they began to understand asylums as important in controlling deviant behaviour.[7] Goffman's influence on the historiography of the asylum is of course paramount. But historians of tuberculosis have been equally impressed by his work and the terminology it offered to study a crucial aspect of tuberculosis management. Linda Bryder has argued in her seminal study of the social history of tuberculosis in Britain that the sanatorium for tuberculosis mostly served social and political functions, as it had little effective therapeutic function. She concluded that the sanatorium is the perfect example of a total institution, as its "real" purpose was discipline and identity formation.[8] Similarly, Sheila Rothman, writing about middle-class experience in the American sanatorium has recognised all the characteristics of total institutions and not much in terms of credible therapeutic success either.[9] Gerd Göckenjan has declared that social control was the only purpose of the sanatorium, as it represented the total failure of medicine's attempts in tuberculo-

sis control before World War II.[10] And finally, Michael Worboys
has conceded that the British sanatorium was more likely to be a
source of cross-infection than a location of effective treatment.[11]

Goffman's notion of a total institution has also helped to encourage historians of tuberculosis to contrast the real-world sanatorium
with the fictional sanatorium, which had dominated the public
imagination of the sanatorium previously and, indeed, had shaped
the early historiographical recognition of this particular medical
institution.[12] The literary sanatorium has been described as a
romantic ocean liner where middle- and upper-class patients are
confined together on a long journey, with ample time for sexual
adventures and philosophical reflections.[13] In many ways, thus, the
total institution, with its emphasis on compulsory re-education and
discipline, is the antithesis par excellence of Thomas Mann's Magic
Mountain. Yet it is my hypothesis in this chapter that historiography has treated Goffman's total institution as the replacement myth
for the Magic Mountain. While the latter has been compared to the
"real world" and found lacking, the notion of the sanatorium as a
total institution itself has never been challenged. It is thus very
tempting to agree with a statement made in 1980: "Goffman is
cited by many, yet examined by few."[14] This chapter aims to change
this, first by challenging the term of the total institution and then by
considering Goffman's other influential writing, on stigma, which
has found equally wide resonance.[15]

GOFFMAN'S TOTAL INSTITUTION AND THE
SANATORIUM FOR TUBERCULOSIS

In order to test the usefulness of Goffman's terminology for the history of the tuberculosis sanatorium, it is of course crucially important to understand the nature of medical institutions in the history
of the disease. Historiography widely agrees that the term "sanatorium for tuberculosis" describes a therapeutic institution available
to patients suffering from tuberculosis that was becoming increasingly popular during the second half of the nineteenth century.[16]
The first sanatorium pioneer, the German physician and 1848 revolutionary activist Dr Hermann Brehmer, opened his sanatorium in
Görbersdorf, Silesia, in 1854 in an abandoned hydrotherapeutic
sanatorium.[17] Led by Brehmer, and later on by his former assistant,
Peter Dettweiler, German sanatorium doctors particularly valued

the open-air rest treatments, where the emphasis was put on remaining outdoors in all weather conditions, coupled with a rich diet. Britain, on the other hand, favored the model of occupational therapy often credited to Marcus Paterson, medical superintendent of the Brompton Hospital Sanatorium at Frimley in Surrey, which opened in 1905.[18] But many other models and mixtures of sanatorium treatment existed: for example, Dr Karl Turban founded the first high-altitude sanatorium in Davos, Switzerland, which combined the establishment of a bacteriological research facility with open-air treatment and regular exercise.[19] A systematic comparative study that took into account a variety of historical contexts, looked at therapeutic regimes, and considered patient experience would be eminently helpful.[20] Suffice to say that it does not seem to be entirely without problems that historians have tended to typecast "the sanatorium" as an ubiquitous and largely stable institution between 1850 and 1950.[21]

Historians of tuberculosis have always been fascinated by the sanatorium. Orthodox accounts of the sanatorium have regarded it as an episode of hospital history and focused on the role of the sanatorium pioneers, such as Hermann Brehmer in Germany, Edward L. Trudeau in the United States, or George Boddington and later Marcus Paterson in Britain.[22] All of them outsiders in one way or another, their histories were told as heroic achievements in the face of adversity. These hagiographic narratives blended in rather nicely with the accounts of later therapeutic innovations, such as the discovery of streptomycin by Selman Waksman and Albert Schatz, which was celebrated as the "conquest of tuberculosis."[23]

Architecture was also regarded as an important element of the sanatorium's master narrative.[24] Indeed, the sanatorium for tuberculosis was one of the main empirical examples that were used to proclaim the study of architecture as a method of choice for historians to link the history of medical theory, practice, and experience.[25] This fascination with the sanatorium's architecture points the way to its wider cultural importance as it caught on with public imagination around the time of World War I.[26] Fictional accounts of the sanatorium, all appearing in a relatively short time span, developed into a remarkable cross-national literary genre, which still remains a somewhat neglected area within the historiography of tuberculosis.[27]

Jean Dubos and René Dubos jumpstarted a social and cultural investigation of the history of tuberculosis with their classic book

The White Plague.[28] Their case highlighted power relations in medicine and discussed tuberculosis as a disease that they understood to
be deeply intertwined with Western culture and society.[29] Linda
Bryder's book, still probably the benchmark study within the social
history of tuberculosis, owes much to the Duboses and goes on to
explicitly argue against the reference model of the Magic Mountain,
as indicated by her choice of title, *Below the Magic Mountain.* Her
main thrust is to understand the political groups and vested interests
behind the anti-tuberculosis movement in England and Wales. Her
chapter on patients explicitly emphasises the usefulness of Goffman,
rather than Mann, for understanding working-class experience in the
sanatorium.[30] If the literary sanatorium has provided the master narrative for middle-class experience in the sanatorium, Goffman's total
institution has been used as a similarly strong paradigm to study
working-class experience in the sanatorium.

The fact that by today's standards sanatorium treatment against
tuberculosis before World War II was comparatively ineffective has
led historians to question its medical merits altogether. Goffman
has stipulated that the given objective of the total institutions – to
treat its patients – ought to be seen as a decoy diverting the attention away from the real goals of the institution. Indeed, growing
medical and political concern about the cost of the sanatorium system, particularly from the 1920s, led the medical superintendents
to move towards an educational, rather than a purely therapeutic, agenda. German doctors sometimes argued that the patients
had to go back to their communities as hygienic apostles, preach-
ing hygiene and moral values to their families and friends.[31] In
Britain, sanatorium advocates initially spoke about "auto-inoculation" through graduated labour treatment, which brought together
preventative, educational, and therapeutic ideas.[32] Historiography has used the educational emphasis as key evidence to deny the
sanatorium the status of an effective medical institution.[33]

But I cannot find this idea of a quasi-conspiracy particularly con-
vincing. Modern, bio-scientifically informed judgments on historical treatments are of limited value.[34] This is evident in the history of
antibiotic treatment against tuberculosis. Here, the close link
between antibiotic effectiveness and the regime of randomised clinical control studies has dramatically restructured the evaluation of
medical success.[35] Against this "gold standard" of tuberculosis
treatment, no previous treatment stands any chance. But such a

statement bears little insight for historians interested in past treatment and its evaluation. Much more fruitfully, rather, can such an interest be explored within a historical, social, and perhaps cultural framing of medical success.[36]

Long before streptomycin and without a universally accepted control regime, success was a complex category indeed. Battles were fought over the stages of tuberculosis before and after treatment and the merits of various methods to measure medical success. While the early twentieth century had become diagnostically capable of a sophisticated bacteriologic analysis, the treatment in the sanatoria in England, Germany, and elsewhere continued to rely on the self-healing proficiencies of the patients. Often only time could tell whether any success had been achieved at all. But doctors, patients, and insurance companies covering the costs asked for immediate results, often after a couple of weeks of therapy. This resulted in a coexistence of incommensurable meanings of therapeutic success. A large proportion of the patients were discharged as "arrested," "improved," or even "healed." It is not clear what kind of clinical assessment was required for any of these discharge diagnoses. Available follow-up records from the Brompton Hospital Sanatorium at Frimley indicate that there was virtually no correlation between discharge diagnosis and length of survival. Indeed, some cases were discharged as "arrested" only to be found dying the very next day. [37]

But there is a further complication for the historical analysis of medical success, as it is not clear that success as a singular concept ever existed. This point can be easily exemplified using tuberculosis therapy as an example. The sanatorium treatment was of course an unspecific intervention against tuberculosis. Most sanatorium doctors were ultimately relatively moderate in their claims, and so was the directly observable outcome. The advocates of sanatorium treatment aimed at raising the probability of survival as the main measurement for success.[38] But at the same time, the funding of sanatorium treatment for the vast majority of patients unable to draw on unlimited private wealth had to be time-limited in order to be cost-effective. Doctors thus had to find criteria to discharge patients even though the long-term likelihood of survival was far from clear.

But what about the patients? Were they to believe that the sanatorium was only marginally important in determining their chances, as the real test was to come afterwards? Or were they better off to just focus on getting out of the sanatorium quite irrespective of their long-term chances? The available sources point to patients clearly reflecting about such conflicting meanings of medical success.[39] One way forward for patients was to take matters into their own hands. Self-diagnosing their health based on linear scales became very popular among patients, as it allowed them to read out any improvement or deterioration in their physical condition. Erich Stern, a medical psychologist and former sanatorium patient himself, observed in 1925 that the patients actually helped the doctors establish these simple scales by constantly debating the results of the "fever curve" and their body weight.[40] The food intake in the sanatorium had a direct influence on the patients' weight and, as such, on their perception of health. Reading and making sense of the latest fever data was of paramount importance for the patients.[41] This constant debate about relative health status supports the idea that the patients played an important role in the *negotiation* of medical success.

The emerging social and welfare policies in Britain and Germany further strengthen the argument in favour of the sanatorium as a multi-functional rather than a one-dimensional institution. The amount of money spent in Britain on tuberculosis treatment in the 1920s was similar to all expenditure on maternity and child welfare services.[42] Only through a complex political process was the sanatorium treatment established as the nearly universal medical answer to the problem of tuberculosis. Historians have successfully challenged the consensus supporting sanatorium treatment, pointing to intense medical controversies around the assessment of medical success.[43] But that just makes the task of explaining the sanatorium's appeal even harder. The available evidence, however, points to the fact that most sanatoria were not generally unpopular institutions amongst patients and, more importantly, the wider community of tuberculosis sufferers. Not only did they offer plenty of food, clean bed linen, and sometimes even the first stay in suburban or rural locations for many, they also promised hope and the potential for successful medical intervention. A useful indicator for this relative popularity is provided by the waiting lists for English sanatoria. Despite some critical remarks about specific sanatoria, such waiting lists for voluntary and state-run sanatoria in England were long and the beds easily filled. In 1930 between two and three thousand patients were on waiting lists for a sanatorium bed in England and Wales at any given time.[44] This appears to bring a category into play that has so far been met with very little historical interest: patient demand.

Clearly, social policy alone would not have sufficed to make the sanatorium into the flagship institution for tuberculosis therapy from 1900. The sanatorium pioneers, often professionally isolated medical doctors, were not important enough to press the issue by themselves, despite setting up more or less successful operations. German critics referred to sanatorium doctors as "nothing else than business-minded hoteliers," and it is doubtful whether they would have been able to promote large-scale sanatorium movements by themselves.[45] The breakthrough on the medical side came with bacteriology. Not only did the shift in medical thought and the ultimate discovery of *mycobacterium tuberculosis* put tuberculosis as an infectious disease on the map after it had been largely ignored by the medical establishment.[46] The subsequent failure of bacteriological attempts at treatment did much to divert the public's attention to other forms of treatment, however basic or non-specific they seemed.[47] Soon after 1891, when Koch's claims to have found an effective treatment against tuberculosis were recognised as overly optimistic, the sanatorium doctors made the case that their institutions should now be seen as the only credible alternative left to provide large-scale treatment.[48] This interplay between patient demand, policy issues, and the production of scientific knowledge is an interesting issue of the *modern* medical marketplace and further undermines the one-term-fits-all approach propagated by Goffman.[49]

SANATORIUM UNDERLIFE: A CASE OF SECONDARY ADAPTATION?

Under the umbrella of the total institution, Goffman has studied a range of issues connected to patients' identity. One of the most original aspects is the analysis of the *hospital underlife*. The idea is that everything the patients can possibly do to make their life in the institution more bearable is essentially stabilizing to the institution, however much the patients act outside the medical authority's approval. Goffman differentiates between primary and secondary adjustment or adaptation. Patients readily spending their afternoons in open-air treatment performed a primary adjustment by doing as told. Patients getting up in the middle of the night to have a chat would be examples of secondary adaptation, as, whilst breaking formal rules of the institution, they would not endanger it. This is where Goffman becomes particularly useful, as his work highlights the importance of studying patients and the way they interact with and contribute to these institutions. For it is only when patients are being studied as legitimate actors – whether within medical instutions or in doctor-patient encounters – that the "patients' view" (Porter) can really be understood.[50] It is thus imperative to overcome the notion that the institution exists independently of its inmates and that patients are mere objects of institutional therapy. Interestingly, this conclusion seems to undermine the theory it is developed from. Indeed, Goffman appears ambiguous about this: on the one hand, the concept of secondary adaptation stimulates the study of patients' experiences and actions, while on the other hand, it denies real agency to the patients. It is therefore still unclear whether or not patients' underlife is mainly to be seen as resistance to or compliance with the aims of the institution.[51]

This issue can be explored further by looking in more detail at the available evidence concerning sanatorium patients. Goffman emphasises implications of long-term institutional confinement and assumes homogeneity of the patients; mobility in the patient population or even changes in its structural composition are not accounted for. The hypothesis to be tested is therefore that a homogenous group of tuberculosis sufferers would more or less show the same behaviour, develop a mutually shared identity whilst in the sanatorium, and possibly retain that shared identity after discharge. Careful analysis of the available sources reveals, however, that virtually none of these criteria were met.[52] To begin with, the social structure in the sanatorium was rather diverse, which regularly led to serious tensions amongst patients. In fact, the case studies suggest that the actual social intake of most sanatoria was fairly diverse. All the tried and tested indicators of patient structure such as age, occupational groups, urban versus rural patients, and even gender composition (in the case of mixed sanatoriums) confirm a heterogeneous patient body.[53]

But what did the patients in these institutions actually do with their time? The signature element offered in most sanatoria in Germany, Britain, and elsewhere was open-air treatment; in other words, exposure to "fresh air" was defined as the prime ingredient of institutional therapy. Relatively large variations occurred between sanatoriums, and certainly between different national sanatorium cultures, as to how this time in the open should be spent.[54] The German model, for example, was based on the idea of long rest hours in open balconies and halls, while the British version ideally took the form of organizing patients to do some outdoor work and/or housekeeping duties with open windows as part of its graduated-labour philosophy.[55]

The German sanatorium, with its emphasis on open-air rest therapy, had its signature element in the large halls where patients stayed during their scheduled rest times. In the more expensive private institutions, they often rested on individual balconies, but the most widespread type of building was the Liegehalle – a south-facing, large, usually roof-covered patio. In Britain, such communal rooms were unusual. Here, open-air therapy was either concentrated in smaller timber huts dispersed around the sanatorium grounds or in wards where patients stayed with windows wide open.

Crucially, though, what virtually all sanatorium systems had in common was that they primarily catered for patients who were still in relatively good health. Indeed, sanatorium doctors tried to ensure that they admitted only treatable patients. Such was this emphasis that there is sound evidence that sanatoria accepted some patients who probably never suffered from tuberculosis at all.[56] Better fed and better rested than at home, sanatorium patients could easily be rather lively and active.[57] It is not surprising, thus, that institutional mortality both in Germany and in Britian was very low. While occasionally patients may have died, any death was usually seen as an accident of institutional management, for when a patient's health deteriorated, the institution usually discharged him or her to a more suitable place of terminal care, such as the home, the workhouse infirmary, or the general hospital.[58]

The relatively healthy sanatorium patients found much joy in social self-organization. Meetings at lunch tables, taking the rest cures together, or even specifically named ward groups provided ample opportunity for this. Such activities helped the patients retain a degree of normality whilst providing entertainment in the unfriendly medical environment. Crucially though, this self-organization had to cater to a relatively dynamic composition of patients. The average time spent in a sanatorium varied considerably from country to country and between different institutions, but treatment cycles usually lasted for several months. This period provided enough time for the patients, who stayed for the duration, to build up and maintain a pretty sophisticated self-organization. Most such organizations show an ambiguous functional structure – independence from and usefulness for the running of the sanatorium.[59]

One such function was the integration of newcomers. Sanatoria were characterized by the nearly constant arrival and departure of patients. Every day, groups of patients left after finishing (or prematurely stopping) their treatment, or arrived to begin their sojourn. This pattern meant that integrating newcomers into medical regimes and social relations presented the sanatorium governors with problems, as there usually was not enough staff to induct fully all the newcomers into the sanatorium. Patient groups had a role to play here. They welcomed the newcomers, gave them a position in a self-regulated club or society, and in such a way helped regulate their behaviour. Whilst patients often spontaneously started such groups as part of a sanatorium's underlife, these self-organizations became essential in maintaining the institutions. They cooperated with the formal authority of the medical staff, and they provided a self-governed form of social control, as they made sure that nobody stepped far out of line. Here is an area of study where Goffman does help to ask the right questions in order to understand the diverse functions of patient self-organization. Whether or not he had any place for an active agency on the part of the patients is perhaps beside the point. What is important is that with the help of Goffman's theories, the "patient's view" can be linked to institutional history.

Romance and sexual encounters between patients make up another much-discussed aspect of patient life in the sanatorium. This point goes back to another classic of patient history, Susan Sontag's much-cited *Illness as Metaphor*, in which she suggested that tuberculosis was a romanticized disease.[60] To the present day there has been surprisingly little discussion about this claim outside the realm of literature analysis. Working-class biographies and what little is known about tuberculosis sufferers certainly do not indicate much romanticism. Medical writers around the time of World War I were already fascinated by the connection between tuberculosis and romantic feelings. Similarly, early-twentieth-century fiction connected the disease with hightened sexual interest.

Thomas Mann and Josef Kessel, to name but two famous writers, have used the sanatorium as the setting for male-female sexual encounters.[61] These fictional accounts are all quite obviously gendered, with their main actors all being male. This pattern suggests a possible connection between disease and masculinity. But all this is strongly based on the sanatorium novel. What, if any, is the relationship between sexual fantasy and actual sexual encounters? This question points to a fundamental methodological problem that can be associated with two classic writers in the field of sexual studies: Michel Foucault emphasised the discourse about sexuality without paying much attention to the "real" sex going on. Alfred C. Kinsey, as an empirical sexologist, was largely focused on counting and classifying sexual encounters as an empirical project.[62] With this in mind, it is clear that sexuality has played an important role in the collective imagination about the sanatorium. But an omnipresence of sex in the sanatorium is at the very least very difficult to substantiate, and where sources confirm such behaviour, it then becomes difficult to judge between the regular and the exceptional.

Historians have usually argued indirectly to build up the plausibility of romanticism and sexuality occurring in the sanatorium. Rothman argues for the United States that patients in mixed sanatoria were aware of their imminent deaths and that, hence, all social regulations were dropped, because everybody lived as fast as possible in the present whilst ignoring the future.[63] This position hinges on the nature of the sanatorium: it seems extremely unlikely that social breakdown would occur within a curative institution, where hope to rejoin the outside world and relatively short sojourns would keep the patients in touch with their social world.[64] The evidence supports this interpretation: social self-organization, noticeable cooperation with staff, and debates about the relative health status of patients do not indicate any breaking down of social regulations and boundaries.

Relationships among staff were not the only option, though weddings between nurses and their patients are well documented, and with the desperate search for nursing and technical staff, sanatoria often appointed former patients, who saw nothing wrong in becoming "familiar with the current patients." Reasons for such feelings or behaviour were manifold. But this hardly ever involved desperation, because life was about to come to an end or a hostile resistance against the sanatorium.[65] In short – romantic feelings, love, and perhaps even sexuality did occur within the sanatorium, but much less as a form of patient underlife or as part of secondary adaptation and much more as a way of linking the sanatorium experience with the outside world too.

PATIENT EXPERIENCE AND THE STIGMA OF TUBERCULOSIS

The analysis of stigma comes from another of Goffman's influential studies.[66] Very much as part of his larger theoretical framework concerned with personal identity, he explored the consequences of stigma, which he primarily conceptualized as damage to the social identity of an individual or a social group. His exploration has implicitly constructed a fairly specific theoretical framework aimed at illuminating the strategies for coping with a stigma, be the latter already visible to others or merely perceived by the bearer.[67] It is thus possible to differentiate between a stigma where discrimination is already taking place and a stigma where the threat of discrimination is merely perceived. However, it is difficult to positively define the variables constituting a stigma. How individual or group characteristics become part of a stigma and what the larger-scale problems of stigma are is not easy to say. In light of recent research on HIV/AIDS and the public health implications of the stigma of disease, history of medicine has an important role to play in providing answers to such questions.[68]

The idea of a link between infectious diseases and fear and blame is of course nothing new. In fact they have been key elements of cultural responses to outbreaks of epidemic diseases at least since the plague epidemics in medieval and early modern Europe.[69] During the cholera epidemics of the 1830s and 1840s, it appears that stigma was readily attached to geographical entities: townships, cities, regions, or countries were seen as centres of epidemic diseases, which had to be avoided at all cost.[70] Through the second half of the century, environmental categories were increasingly replaced by social ones, as the industrial working classes became identified with disease.[71] It might thus be argued that tuberculosis became increasingly associated with social problems precisely when germ theory emerged to conceptualise the disease as a communicable, rather than a constitutional, disease. This argument provides an important insight for the history of tuberculosis, because it pits advocates of the stigma of tuberculosis directly against Susan Sontag's notion of a romanticized representation of tuberculosis.[72] My purpose is, however, not to investigate the stigma of tuberculosis in its entirety but, rather, to focus on the interdependence of medical institutions and the production of stigma. This has not received enough attention because of the historiographical emphasis on boundaries between the institution and the wider society, as exemplified by the total institution. Stigma was conceptualised as happening outside of and independently of institutions. As one of the results of the analysis so far is to see a much weaker separation between institutions and society, it is only plausible to extend the focus now to examine the stigma *and* the medical institution.

Let us begin again with the familiar tuberculosis novel. The literary stigma understood as the loss of social identity, for example in Mann's *Magic Mountain* or Kessler's *Les Captifs,* centred around the time of absence from society.[73] While the duration of the fictional cures bears little resemblance to real-world experiences of sanatorium treatment, these novels use time very effectively to link the sanatorium world with the rest of society. The absence from regular social life is crafted as in itself suspicious and as an indication that the protagonists suffer from tuberculosis. This fictional conceptualization of stigma hinges on the social valuation of time and place. Once the sanatorium was firmly established, prolonged absence could easily be perceived as suspicious, regardless of one's physical condition, and, to a degree, it could replace the appearance of physical signs of illness. In fact, the literary patient often contrasts healthy looks with disease histories. Duration of absence and physical appearance could thus send conflicting messages. I suggest understanding the social value of time as a crucial element when attempting to understand the implications of sanatorium treatment for non-fictional patients. Historical studies of urban mobility in German cities confirm the intense intra-urban mobility: a substantial proportion of working-class households changed addresses within a twelve-month period.[74] Being away for several months to get treatment in a sanatorium, therefore, implied coming back to a changed world: friends might have moved, or the patient's family itself might have moved. One former patient who was treated in Frimley sanatorium near London before World War II described the situation: "My main interest was of course the cinema, of which I had always been fond, but became increasingly addicted to for it was indeed a lonely time for me. We had moved house while I had been away and I had again completely lost touch with my friends."[75]

This loss of social life owing to prolonged absence struck relatively young and unmarried patients particularly hard. And for many patients sanatorium treatment was not a one-off experience, since many went through treatment cycles as they were often readmitted or passed on to different sanatoriums. This cycle was a consequence of social policy, because the duration of each round of treatment was limited by cost. The underlying economic principle suggested that any treatment was viable provided that it restored a patient sufficiently to permit participation in the labour market again. If such restoration lasted long enough, another round of sanatorium treatment was justifiable.[76] This institutional cycle resulted in real struggles for the patients. Moritz Bromme, a German worker who was a patient at the Charlottenhöhe sanatorium near Stuttgart before World War I, returned to his family after treatment. Since the industrial labour market was offering opportunities for skilled workers, he soon found work even though everybody understood the industrial conditions to be at least partly responsible for his disease. Consequently, every minor cold was interpreted as a clear sign of disease progression. "But what now? That was the big question. I finally ended up in an industrial factory again, that was the sad end of all my treatment. After one month, I had contracted a bad influenza and [had] to call in sick. My foreman asked me 'How long this time? – I bet you end up in the Castle of the Coughers within a year!'"[77]

In this example, the regularity of a prolonged absence is at the basis of lay knowledge about tuberculosis and points to a common understanding of the inability to cure. The disease, mediated through the sanatorium cures, clearly kept Bromme from achieving social mobility. His well-founded aspirations for leaving the factory job were rendered hopeless because of his disease, which in turn cannot have benefited from the working conditions in the factory. This led to a vicious cycle of going back and forth between sanatorium and factory, while his family had to endure considerable hardship. Every time Moritz went to the sanatorium, his wife and children faced extreme poverty. Without a wage earner around and being forced to look after five young children, his wife was as much the target of stigmatization as Moritz himself. He blamed himself and his disease for leaving his family vulnerable, and he felt guilt about the relative generosity of sanatorium life compared to the hardships his family had to endure.[78]

If the stigma of tuberculosis meant the loss of social identity because of the disease, then no longer being capable of supporting a family at a relatively young age ranked equally highly on the scale of intimidating factors. Of course, this problem did not go unnoticed by the organizers of sanatorium treatment. While the National Insurance Act in Britain did not provide for families and relied on local poor relief to support dependants, the German health insurance system entered an agreement with the Imperial Insurance Office to provide for family members of sanatorium patients treated under the governance of the invalid insurance.[79] However, while this provision indicates that, at least in Germany, policy-makers accepted the problem, the proposed solution did relatively little to solve it. Sanatorium treatment may itself have been perfectly respectable, but it often implied that the family had to apply for poor relief, which in turn could well have led to a loss of social status.[80]

Orthodox sanatorium treatment did occasionally interfere directly with patients' bodies through cold-water showers, medical examinations, and wrapping patients up in blankets. Some institutions even employed dedicated staff who concentrated on wrapping them up as tightly as possible. This treatment certainly regulated physical activities and hygienic behavior within the institution very explicitly. But the regime was limited to the sanatorium, and it was largely up to the patients to carry the experience into their lives after discharge.[81] The adoption of chest surgery as a routine treatment for tuberculosis in the 1920s changed this. Invasive medical treatment implied a metamorphosis of the body that changed the long-term implications of treatment considerably. Chest surgery was introduced to tuberculosis treatment before World War I, following the pioneering work by Carlo Forlanini in 1888. The driving forces behind German chest surgery in 1920 were innovations in practice, the growing importance of surgery in clinical practice, and the change of the sanatorium into a specialist chest hospital. Chest surgery changed the doctor-patient relationship in the sanatorium. Doctors often saw these operations as honorable for the patients. Dr Fred Holmes, a u.s. surgeon, wrote in 1935 that chest surgery results in a "medal to be pinned on the battle-scarred veteran after a bloody campaign."[82] The price to pay for this medal was, however, high from the point of view of the patient. Jack, a Swiss working-class patient at the Zurich alpine sanatorium in Clavadel, wrote in a letter to his sister:

> Thursday morning, at 11 o'clock, I was prepared to get my nerves squeezed. Normally this procedure takes up half an hour. Well, I was comfortable in my beddings and covered from head to toe, only my throat was free. Before getting covered, I had seen the doctors, all dressed in white with only the eyes uncovered. The narcotics started to have an effect and I didn't feel much of all the butchery until some complications occured. After that, I had to feel exactly how many nerves there are in me. I'd rather go to the dentist to have three nerves extracted than endure another operation of my chest.[83]

Because chest surgery was widely used as a treatment for far-advanced cases, Jack, not unlike many other patients who underwent chest surgery, died within a couple of weeks of the operation.[84]

One reason for the popularity of chest surgery was that it was easy to perform and required only basic operating equipment. Also, the procedure put surgery successfully on the map in the control of tuberculosis, the single most important cause of adult death. With this change from an unspecific institutional to a specialist treatment came a change in the way medical success was studied, as it became legitimate to note a patient's survival without any follow-up concerns.[85] For the doctors, the intervention quickly became routine; for patients, however, it was usually the first experience with surgery and the modern hospital environment, which fundamentally changed the treatment experience. With sanatorium patients often consumed by a lay interpretation of medical information, for example, by body temperature or weight, it is interesting to note that surgery patients gained in social status through the medical intervention. Going through a painful operation and living to tell the story was seen as a sign of true grit – and in lay medical terms this was the most important requirement for beating tuberculosis. The "battle medal" was reflected by the patients, as they regarded those who had endured heavy surgery to be the veterans. This internal hierarchy according to medical procedure could best develop in an environment where patients stayed for prolonged periods. One English patient reported later on that "curious medical snobberies arose out of these treatments. Thoracoplastic cases looked down unchallenged from the height of their surgical experience ... As I wheeled through the corridor-lounge the walking patients were just returning from their morning stroll. They smiled and patted my legs, and I felt like giving the double handshake with which heavy-weight boxers greet their fans after a knockout. Triumph was mine."[86]

A strong gender component is present in accounts of heroism and surgery, though. Generally, documents from women about treatment for tuberculosis are more skeptical.[87] Female patients confirmed that chest surgery was an intimidating experience, but they did not report any change of status in the informal hierarchy among the patients. Pride about physical pain experienced seems to have been a sign of masculinity, while women were simply expected to comply. But for men, surviving operations raised them into the "aristocracy of tuberculosis".[88] However, on discharge from the sanatorium, the consequences of surgery resulted in a distinct change in this perception, because chest surgery then endangered masculinity. Within the sanatorium, the apparent physical disability was a bonus for men, but outside this currency became invalid, since the social and psychological identity of the patient was permanently damaged. An English middle-class patient reported of his life after chest surgery: "Another of my difficulties was the problem of women standing in buses and trains. If I remained seated I felt uncomfortable and loutish, and if I stood I suffered real pain as the vehicle rattled and jolted ... What I did was to travel a little later when the buses and trains were less crowded ... I have evolved countless ways of keeping myself out of difficulty."[89]

His strategy was to avoid most social contacts, and he did so because he felt his body was inadequate to participate in social life as a normal man. It is remarkable to note that his worst feelings had to do with general courtesy to women, which makes the gendered nature of chest surgery and its longer-term implications very obvious. For those surgery patients who lived long enough, life after medical treatment was often a lonely one precisely because of what had happened in the institution. Another patient described such immediate problems: "My doctor was in no hurry for me to go back to work and I was content not to do so, for I had developed a giant-sized inferiority complex. I had all the usual youthful desires, but felt I was a social outcast as far as girls were concerned. So, it was the heroines of the Cinema I courted, rescuing them from impossible situations and seducing them in their eternal gratitude of my heroic exploits."[90]

The long-term effects of chest surgery, however challenging for masculinity, affected not only men of course, since chest surgery led to disabled bodies regardless of gender. The change from a comparatively healthy body to a disabled body happened in the institution. But how this change then played out in practice was clearly gendered, as was the whole experience of sanatorium treatment. Without the option to become a "veteran patient," women often felt more strongly about the sanatorium and became rather more alienated by this institution. One woman who was treated in an English sanatorium directly after World War II noticed that "actually coping with everyday tasks with a collapsed lung was a trial, but it was a joy to be away from the suffocating atmosphere of the sanatorium."[91] She further noted how much the inhabitants of her former social surroundings withdrew from her, thinking that she was still a threat to their health. Interestingly, she reported on the combined effects of her physical absence, which was clearly noted in her community, as well as on the relation between disability through tuberculosis and a loss of social identity: "Rehabilitation to normal life, including overcoming social prejudices, was prolonged, pride enabled me to persevere with the painful exercises needed to restore my now deformed right side to some degree of normality but it was many years before I was brave enough to wear a swimsuit."[92]

This story points to an important element in the history of chest surgery: medical intimidation. Reading patients' accounts in the light of our knowledge of the absence of any regulated medical quality control shows that operations could become instruments of power for the surgeons involved. The sources reveal patients who initially accepted the operations and follow-up interventions but later on in their lives refused to comply. That reaction is not entirely surprising, since chest surgery often contributed to prolonged medical problems. Recent years have seen renewed interest in chest surgery for the treatment of drug-resistant cases. At the same time, there is still a perceived danger of the dissemination of tuberculosis by former patients of chest surgery of the 1930s and 1940s, which has reminded the medical community of the long-term consequences of medical treatment.[93] In the strictest sense of the term, the effects of the stigma suffered by chest tuberculosis patients was more a consequence of the medical intervention than of the disease itself. This confirms the hypothesis that the institution and the treatment therein were fundamentally related to the long-term consequences for the patients outside the institution.

CONCLUSION

Goffman's work has been very persuasive in drawing attention to the situation of patients and inmates in long-term institutional confinement. His *Asylums* was linked with a range of critical accounts of modern psychiatry and contributed substantially to a shift in the sociology of madness, which in turn has been instrumental in enriching the historiography of the asylum. Similarly, historians of tuberculosis have found Goffman useful in studying the sanatorium. The concept of the total institution has served as a focus point for working-class experience in medical institutions and, specifically in the history of tuberculosis, has developed into an icon for the critical stance that social history has taken towards the sanatorium. On closer inspection, however, it appears that the concept of the total institution can be reformulated into a set of empirically significant assumptions. Put to the test, the concept then loses much of its attraction.

The main argument against the concept of the total institution relates to the problem of medical success. The historiography of tuberculosis has perhaps underestimated the historical nature of the term itself. Pointing to the usefulness or redundant nature of any past medical treatment is problematic. But in the case of tuberculosis, where effective medication became available after World War II, most historians have not been able to resist measuring previous treatment regimes against the success of antibiotics. Historians should perhaps be sceptical about the "truth about antibiotics," given the struggles with resistance and overprescription of such medication.[94] But it appears to be an ill-advised strategy to use a contemporary treatment as the point of reference for past treatment, because it is in the very nature of medical success for it to be framed as a historical rather than an absolute category.

Where inspired by Goffman, it has been argued that the sanatorium was an ineffective institution. This chapter has proposed to reconsider the sanatorium and its medical success in light of the historical framing of disease and its treatment.

Goffman's concept of secondary adjustment is a particularly intriguing idea. While connected to the total institution concept, it highlights the importance of studying patients in medical institutions in all their activities. Thus, patients' own activities must be seen within a wider framework. Goffman's answer, that whatever patients do they ultimately help to stabilize the institution, has been shown wanting. If the sanatorium is a multi-functional setup, then the multi-functionality must be true for patients' activities no less. They might have worked together with the institution, possibly even stabilising an otherwise dynamic setting through maintaining a sense of normality. Yet this was orientated towards their outside world as much as they contributed to an important task within the sanatorium.

All this is not to say that the total institution is a completely redundant concept. In fact, by working against its many assumptions and using it as a Weberian ideal-type, we find that it almost counterfactually supports the analysis of the sanatorium as a multi-functional institution. Not only does it become rather clear that different groups identified different functions with the sanatorium, it is also increasingly evident that patients' opinions about the sanatorium were far from unified. Clearly, the wider institutional context played a major role, as did the history of the sanatorium itself. The arrival of chest surgery, for example, changed the patient experience in the sanatorium quite dramatically. This is where Goffman's writings on stigma become very helpful, for it is this term that allows us to tie the sanatorium to the outside world. One of the major weaknesses of most theories of medical institutions is that they either stop or start at the hospital gate. The total institution is no exception to this statement, as it keeps the purpose of the sanatorium firmly within its walls. Examining the stigma of tuberculosis in relation to institutional treatment overcomes this limitation. Any future analysis of the stigma of tuberculosis will have to take into account that the loss of social identity may well have been more heavily influenced by the institutional set-up than by the disease alone.

Goffman's theories taken at face value deserve revision. His ideas show their age and sound too *Cold War* with their emphasis on identity and compulsory re-education. The available sanatorium case studies confirm that they were no concentration camps; equally they were no cosy Magic Mountains either. If, however, Goffman serves as an inspiration to look at the sanatorium in a fresh way, then he might still be an inspiration for the historiography of medical institutions.

NOTES

1 Erving Goffman, *Asylums: Essays on the Social Situation of Mental Patients and Other Inmates* (New York: Doubleday 1961, 1991).

2 Thomas Szasz, *The Myth of Mental Illness: Foundations of a Theory of Personal Conduct* (New York: Paul B. Hoeber 1961).

3 Ivan Illich, *Medical Nemesis: The Expropriation of Health* (New York: Pantheon 1976).

4 Ludmilla Jordanova, "The Social Construction of Medical Knowledge," *Social History of Medicine* 8 (1995): 361–81.

5 Kathleen Jones and A.J. Fowles, *Ideas on Institutions: Analysing the Literature on Long-Term Care and Custody* (London: Routledge, Keegan and Paul 1984), 9–26.

6 Goffman, *Asylums*, 11.

7 David Rothman, *The Discovery of the Asylum* (Boston, MA: De Gruyter 1971); Andrew Scull, *Museums of Madness: The Social Organisation of Insanity in Nineteenth-Century England* (London: Allan Lane 1979); Elaine Showalter, *The Female Malady: Women, Madness and English Culture, 1830–1980* (New York: Pantheon 1985).

8 Linda Bryder, *Below the Magic Mountain: A Social History of Tuberculosis in Twentieth-Century Britain* (Oxford: Clarendon Press 1988), 200.

9 Sheila M. Rothman, *Living in the Shadow of Death: Tuberculosis and the Social Experience of Illness in American History* (New York: Basic 1994), 227.

10 Gert Göckenjan, *Kurieren und Staat machen: Gesundheit und Medizin in der bürgerlichen Welt* (Frankfurt a. M.: Fischer-TB 1985), 54.

11 Michael Worboys, "The Sanatorium Treatment for Consumption in Britain, 1890–1914," in John V. Pickstone (ed.), *Medical Innovations in Historical Perspective* (New York: Palgrave MacMillan 1992), 47–71.

12 Axel H. Murken, "Vom Heilpalast zum Sanatorium des Volkes," *Die Waage* 21 (1982): 64–72.

13 Vera Pohland, *Das Sanatorium als literarischer Ort: Medizinische Institution und Krankheit als Medien der Gesellschaftskritik und Existenzanalyse* (Frankfurt a. M.: Peter Lang 1984).

14 Jason Ditton (ed.), *The View from Goffman* (London: MacMillan 1980), 13.

15 Erving Goffman, *Stigma* (Englewood Cliffs, NJ: Prentice-Hall 1963).

16 See the references in Flurin Condrau, "Urban Tuberculosis Patients and Sanatorium Treatment in the Early Twentieth Century," in Anne Borsay and Peter Shapely (eds.), *Medicine, Charity and Mutual Aid: The Consumption of Health and Welfare, c.1550–1950* (Aldershot: Ashgate 2007), 183–206.

17 Ingeborg Langerbeins, *Lungenheilanstalten in Deutschland von 1854–1945* (Köln: Diss. med 1979).

18 Marcus S. Paterson, "Graduated Labour in Pulmonary Tuberculosis," *Lancet* 86 (1908, I): 216–20; Marcus S. Paterson, *Auto-Inoculation in Pulmonary Tuberculosis* (London: Nisbet 1911).

19 Karl Turban, *Beiträge zur Kenntnis der Lungentuberkulose* (Wiesbaden: J.F. Bergmann 1899).

20 Flurin Condrau, "Lungenheilstätten im internationalen Vergleich: Zur Sozialgeschichte der Tuberkulose im 19. und frühen 20. Jahrhundert," *Historia Hospitalium* 19 (1993/1994): 220–34.

21 Flurin Condrau, "The Institutional Career of Tuberculosis Patients in Britain and Germany," in John Henderson, Peregrine Horden, and Alessandro Pastore (eds.), *The Impact of Hospitals in Europe, 1000–2002* (Oxford: Peter Lang 2007), 327–57.

22 J. Harley Williams, *Requiem for a Great Killer: The Story of Tuberculosis* (London: Health Horizon 1973).

23 Salman A. Waksman, *The Conquest of Tuberculosis* (Berkeley: University of California Press 1964); Frank Ryan, *Tuberculosis: The Greatest Story Never Told* (Bromsgrove: Swift 1992).

24 Murken, "Vom Heilpalast zum Sanatorium des Volkes"; Axel Hinrich Murken "Heilanstalten für Tuberkulöse: Zur Geschichte der Lungensanatorien und ihrer Therapiekonzeption im 19. Jahrhundert," in W. Göpfert and H.-H. Otten (eds.), *Metanoeite: Wandelt euch durch neues Denken. Festschrift für Professor Hans Schadewaldt zur Vollendung des 60. Lebensjahres* (Düsseldorf: Triltsch 1983), 107–24.

25 Dieter Jetter, *Grundzüge der Krankenhausgeschichte, 1800–1900* (Darmstadt: Wissenschaftliche Buchgesellschaft 1977).

26 Margaret Campbell, "What Tuberculosis Did for Modernism: The Influence of a Curative Environment on Modernist Design and Architecture," *Medical History* 49 (2005): 463–88.

27 See Pohland, *Das Sanatorium als literarischer Ort*.

28 René Dubos and Jean Dubos, *The White Plague: Tuberculosis, Man and Society* (Boston: Little Brown 1952, 1987).

29 As the most consequent "Dubosian" historian see Katherine Ott, *Fevered Lives: Tuberculosis in American Culture since 1870* (Cambridge, MA: Harvard University Press 1996).

30 Bryder, *Below the Magic Mountain*, 199–226.

31 O. Roepke, "Tuberkulose und Heilstätte," *Beiträge zur Klinik der Tuberkulose* 3 (1904):15.

32 Paterson, *Auto-Inoculation in Pulmonary Tuberculosis*.

33 Göckenjan, *Kurieren*, 54.

34 Charles E. Rosenberg and Janet Golden (eds.), *Framing Disease: Studies in the Cultural History* (New Brunswick: Rutgers University Press 1992), xiii–xxvi.

35 Sunil Amrith, "In Search of a Magic Bullet for Tuberculosis: South India and Beyond, 1955–1965," *Social History of Medicine* 17 (2004): 113–30; Helen Valier and Carsten Timmermann, "Clinical Trials and the Reorganization of Medical Research in post-Second World War Britain," *Medical History* 52 (2008): 493–510.

36 Condrau, "Urban Tuberculosis Patients and Sanatorium Treatment in the Early Twentieth Century."

37 Flurin Condrau, "Behandlung ohne Heilung: Zur sozialen Konstruktion des Behandlungserfolgs bei Tuberkulose im frühen 20. Jahrhundert," *Medizin, Gesellschaft und Geschichte* XIX (Stuttgart: Steiner 2001), 71–93.

38 Peter Dettweiler, "Einige Bemerkungen zur sogenannten Ruhe- und Luftliegekur bei Schwindsüchtigen," *Zeitschrift für Tuberkulose und Heilstättenwesen* 1 (1900): 96–100, 180–7.

39 Moritz W.T. Bromme, *Lebensgeschichte eines modernen Fabrikarbeiters* (Jena: Diederichs 1905).

40 Erich Stern, *Die Psyche des Lungenkranken: Der Einfluß der Lungentuberkulose und des Sanatoriumslebens* (Halle: Marhold 1925).

41 Michael Martin, "Bedeutung und Funktion des medizinischen Messens in geschlossenen Patienten-Kollektiven: Das Beispiel der Lungensanatorien," in Volker Hess (ed.), *Normierung der Gesundheit: Messende Verfahren der Medizin als kulturelle Praktik um 1900* (Husum: Matthiesen 1997), 145–64.

42 F.B. Smith, "Review of Below the Magic Mountain by Linda Bryder," *Medical History* 33 (1989): 267.

43 Worboys, *Sanatorium*.

44 Quarterly Returns on Form T.52c, Tuberculosis Files of the Ministry of Health, National Archives, MH 55.144.

45 Franz Wehmer, "Rückblick auf Brehmers Lebensarbeit," *Beiträge zur Klinik der Tuberkulose* 31 (1914): 460.

46 J. Arthur Myers, *Captain of All These Men of Death: Tuberculosis Historical Highlights* (St Louis, MO: Warren Green 1977).

47 Christoph Gradmann, "A Harmony of Illusions: Clinical and Experimental Testing of Robert Koch's Tuberculin 1890–1900," *Studies in History and Philosophy of Biological and Biomedical Sciences*, 34c (2003): 465–81.

48 Christoph Gradmann, "Robert Koch and the Pressures of Scientific Research: Tuberculosis and Tuberculin," *Medical History* 45 (2001): 1–32.

49 Ilana Löwy, "Trustworthy Knowledge and Desperate Patients: Clinical Tests for New Drugs from Cancer to AIDS," in Margaret Lock, Allan Young, and Alberto Cambrosio (eds.), *Living and Working with the New Medical Technologies* (Cambridge: Cambridge University Press 2000).

50 Roy Porter, "The Patient's View: Doing Medical History from Below," *Theory and Society* 14 (1985): 175–98.

51 Jeremy A. Greene, "Therapeutic Infidelities: 'Noncompliance' Enters the Medical Literature, 1955–1975," *Social History of Medicine* 17 (2004): 327–43.

52 Flurin Condrau, *Lungenheilanstalt und Patientenschicksal: Sozialgeschichte der Tuberkulose in Deutschland und England im späten 19. und frühen 20. Jahrhundert* (Göttingen: Vandenhoeck und Ruprecht 2000), 165–212.

53 Flurin Condrau, "Die Patienten von Lungenheilanstalten, 1890–1930: Deutschland und England im Vergleich," in Alfons Labisch and Reinhard Spree (eds.), *Von der Armenfürsorge zur kommunalen Dienstleistung: Finanzwirtschaft und Patienten Allgemeiner Krankenhäuser in Deutschland während des 19. und frühen 20. Jahrhunderts* (Frankfurt a.M.: Campus 2001), 427–48.

54 Condrau, "Lungenheilstätten im internationalen Vergleich."

55 Condrau, *Lungenheilanstalt und Patientenschicksal*, 119–64.

56 Katja Mann seems never to have suffered from tuberculosis. See for details Christian Virchow, *Medizinhistorisches um den "Zauberberg": "Das gläserne Angebinde" und ein pneumologisches Nachspiel* (Augsburg: Universität Augsburg 1995); Philip Ellman, *Chest Disease in General Practice with Special Reference to Pulmonary TB* (London: Lewis 1932), 164.

57 Stern, *Psyche.*

58 Condrau, "The Institutional Career of Tuberculosis."

59 Flurin Condrau, "Who Is the Captain of All These Men of Death? The Social Structure of TB Sanatorium Patients in Postwar Germany," *Journal of Interdisciplinary History* 32 (2001): 243–62.

60 Susan Sontag, *Illness as Metaphor* (New York 1978).

61 Thomas Mann, *Der Zauberberg* (Berlin: Fischer 1924, English 1927); Joseph Kessel, *Les Captifs* (Paris 1926).

62 Michel Foucault, *Histoire de la Sexualité*, 3 vols. (Paris Gallimard 1976–1984, English from 1978); Alfred C. Kinsey, Wardell B. Pomeroy, and Clyde E. Martin, *Sexual Behaviour in the Human Male* (Philadelphia: Saunders 1948).

63 Rothman, *Living in the Shadow of Death.*

64 Condrau, "The Institutional Career of Tuberculosis."

65 Bryder, *Below the Magic Mountain*, 212–14.

66 Goffman, *Stigma*, 12.

67 Vera Das, "Stigma, Contagion, Defect: Issues in the Anthropology of Public Health," *Stigma and Global Health: Developing a Research Strategy* (Bethesda: NIH 2001): http://www.stigmaconference.nih.gov/DasPaper.htm.

68 Jeanine Cogan and Gregory Herek, "Stigma," in Raymond A. Smith (ed.), *Encyclopedia of AIDS: A Social, Political, Cultural, and Scientific Record of the HIV Epidemic* (Chicago: Fitzroy Dearborn 1998), 466–7; Gregory M. Herek, "Illness, Stigma, and AIDS," in Paul T. Costra Jr and Gary R. VandenBos (eds.), *Psychological Aspects of Serious Illness: Chronic Conditions, Fatal Diseases, and Clinical Care* (Washington, DC: American Psychological Association 1990).

69 Peter Baldwin, *Contagion and the State in Europe, 1830–1930* (Cambridge: Cambridge University Press 1999).

70 Erwin H. Ackerknecht, "Anticontagionism between 1821 and 1867," *Bulletin of the History of Medicine* 22 (1948): 562–93; Christopher Hamlin, "Predisposing Causes and Public Health in Early Nineteenth-Century Medical Thought," *Social History of Medicine* 5 (1992): 43–70.

71 John V. Pickstone "Ferrier's Fever to Kay's Cholera: Disease and Social Structure in Cottonopolis," *History of Science* 22 (1984): 401–19.

72 See Bryder, *Below the Magic Mountain*; Ott, *Tuberculosis*; Sontag, *Illness as Metaphor.*

73 Mann, *Zauberberg*; Kessel, *Les Captifs.*

74 Stephan Bleek, "Mobilität und Seßhaftigkeit in deutschen Großstädten während der Urbanisierung," *Geschichte und Gesellschaft* 15 (1989): 5–33.

75 George A. Cook, *A Hackney Memory Chest* (London: Centreprise Trust 1983), 68.

76 Condrau, "The Institutional Career of Tuberculosis."

77 Bromme, *Lebensgeschichte eines modernen Fabrikarbeiters*, 342.

78 Ibid., 295.

79 Ludwig Teleky, "Die Bekämpfung der Tuberkulose," in Adolf Gottstein et al. (eds.), *Handbuch der sozialen Hygiene und Gesundheitsfürsorge*, vol. 3 (Berlin: Springer 1926), 207–341.

80 Sylvelyn Hähner-Rombach, *Sozialgeschichte der Tuberkulose: Vom Kaiserreich bis zum Ende des Zweiten Weltkriegs unter besonderer Berücksichtigung Württembergs* (Stuttgart: Steiner 2000), 186.

81 O. Kuthy, "Erfahrungen über die hygienisch-erzieherische Wirkung der Lungenheilstätten: Aus dem Königin Elisabeth-Sanatorium bei Budapest," *Zeitschrift für Tuberkulose* 9 (1906): 449–56.

82 Fred Holmes, *Tuberculosis: A Book for the Patient* (New York: Appleton-Century 1935), 283f.

83 Jack, letter to his sister, made available to me by Dr Iris Ritzmann, Medizinhistorisches Institut, University of Zurich.

84 Iris Ritzmann, *Hausordnung und Liegekur: Vom Volkssanatorium zur Spezialklinik; 100 Jahre Zürcher Höhenklinik Wald* (Zürich: Chronos 1998).

85 Hertha Liebe, "Kritischer Bericht über 104 Pneumothoraxfälle," *Beiträge zur Klinik der Tuberkulose* 49 (1921): 125–37.

86 Alan Dick, *A Walking Miracle* (London 1942), 68, 95.

87 Flurin Condrau, "Frauen in Lungenheilanstalten zu Beginn des 20. Jahrhunderts in Deutschland und England," in Ulrike Lindner and Merith Niehuss (eds.), *Ärztinnen – Patientinnen: Frauen im deutschen und britischen Gesundheitswesen des 20 Jahrhunderts* (Köln: Böhlau 2002), 199–214.

88 Dick, *Miracle*, 47.

89 Ibid., 129f.

90 Ibid.

91 Joan McCarthy, "'Tuberculosis' before and after Waksman," unpublished BA thesis, Chester College, 1986, 44.

92 Ibid., 45.

93 E. Kniehl et. al., "Rupture of Therapeutic Oleothorax Leading to Paraffin Oil Aspiration and Dissemination of Tuberculosis – A Fatal Late Complication of Tuberculosis Therapy in the 1940s," *Wiener Klinische Wochenschrift* 110 (1998): 725–8; M. Teschner, "Chirurgie von Spätkomplikationen einer ehemals stattgefundenen aktiven Behandlung

der Lungentuberkulose mittels extrapleuraler Plombeneinlage,"
Pneumologie 52 (1998): 115–20; P. Hollaus et al., "Oleothorax: Die
Bombe aus der Vergangenheit tickt weiter (editorial)," *Wiener Klinische
Wochenschrift* 110 (1998): 697f.

94 "Tracking Down the Truth about Antibiotics," Scarborough, Whitby &
Ryedale Primary Care Trust, Press Release 05/197, http://www.swr-pcg.
nhs.uk/news/Associated_Documents/PR197%20-%20Moxy%20Malone.
pdf (30/5/2006).

5

The Great White Plague Turns Alien: Tuberculosis and Immigration in Australia, 1901–2001

ALISON BASHFORD

INTRODUCTION

The historiography of modern nationalism has recently taken a distinct turn. A number of studies have shown how the public health management of populations through medico-legal border control has actively constituted national identities. And many of these studies have persuasively demonstrated the close connections between communicable-disease prevention, race-based exclusions and restrictions, and the formation of racialised nations.[1] Australian history is exemplary in this respect, in large part because of the stridency and efficacy of the white Australia policy. Initially implemented in each of the Australasian colonies in the late nineteenth century, the national Immigration Restriction Act (1901) was one version of the Chinese exclusion acts then proliferating across the globe. Elsewhere I have detailed the extent to which race-based immigration restriction was technically and legally (as well as rhetorically and culturally) part of Australia's public health policy in the early and mid-twentieth-century.[2] In this chapter, and against this historical and historiographical background, I trace Australian medico-legal border control with respect to tuberculosis over the entire twentieth century: that is, from the establishment of the new Australian nation – the Commonwealth of Australia – in 1901 to the crises of border protection, nationally and internationally, at the end of 2001. In 1901 tuberculosis simply did not register as a communicable disease requiring quarantine or immigration regulation. Unlike leprosy or smallpox, it had nothing to do with the racialised pollution anxiety that in large part rationalised the invention and implementation of the white Australia policy. In 2001, however, tuberculosis was the one and only disease for which people were denied a visa or entry into Australia.

This dramatic shift overarches complicated and intersecting lines of Australian migration and public health history, as well as the natural history of the disease. I trace the changing epidemiology of tuberculosis from endemic high morbidity in 1901 to very low morbidity in the overall national population in 2001. I am interested also in the accompanying shift in cultural comprehension of the disease from being the "the great white plague" affecting most families in the country, white as well as Indigenous, to being a disease almost exclusively associated with refugees and migrants. Finally, I map these shifts in tuberculosis epidemiology and comprehension within the changing patterns of migration in twentieth-century Australia, from predominantly British migration under the white Australia policy to the incorporation of Southern and Eastern European migrants in large numbers after the Second World War, and since the mid-1970s, people from Southeast Asia and the Middle East.

From the mid-1970s onwards, tuberculosis has been increasingly linked rhetorically, but also epidemiologically, with refugees and migrants. In more and less explicit ways, this link has been articulated with recourse to the conflation of race, disease, and "invasion," which characterised the early white Australia policy and the Immigration Restriction Act. In the early twentieth century, the threat and prevention of tuberculosis was often conceptualised similarly to the "invading" "Chinese" diseases of nineteenth- century Australia: leprosy and smallpox.[3] But tracing this resurgence of racialised discourse alone would be too easy: doing so would simultaneously reproduce the problematic image of the diseased "coloured alien" so constantly discussed in Australian history and obscure the common problematising of other groups and other factors. In particular, I pay historical attention to the ways in which British migration to Australia was also scrutinised and bureaucratised over the twentieth century. Furthermore, while offering a critique of the return of the "Asian invasion" narrative through the refugee-tuberculosis scare from the late 1990s, it would be a sleight of hand to ignore the epidemiological data. Rather than dismissing public articulations about tuberculosis and global refugee and migrant movement as simply racist (a common but not necessarily the most thoughtful move), I incorporate into this historical and cultural analysis, data that clearly shows higher incidence amongst asylum-seekers and refugees, both from Southeast Asia and more recently from the Middle East.

Thus, in this chapter I trace the (racialised) shift from an endemic great white plague in the first half of the twentieth century to the conceptualisation of tuberculosis as a thoroughly alien disease. But I want to complicate this historical story as well. The chapter proceeds chronologically, surveying first the emergence of linked immigration and quarantine measures that were a central part of white Australia and its "coloured alien" exclusions. I then discuss the period between 1901 and 1948, when "white Australia" was thoroughly and endemically infected with tuberculosis. In this period, health screening of Britons was implemented with ever-increasing reference to tuberculosis. From 1948 until 1976 a large-scale National Prevention Campaign reduced morbidity and mortality in the white population dramatically, and this coincided with a new focus on tuberculous migrants from postwar Europe, as well as British assisted migrants. In the final section, I discuss the coincident abandonment of the National Prevention Campaign in 1976 with the sudden increase in refugees from Southeast Asia in that very year.

"THE VIRGIN CONTINENT": IMMIGRATION, HEALTH SCREENING, AND "WHITE AUSTRALIA"

In the late nineteenth century, the Australian colonies, like many other places in the world, hosted a virulently anti-Chinese culture. Chinese people had entered the country initially with the mid-nineteenth-century goldrushes. Even though white culture and governance itself constituted an alien invasion, having been on the continent only two or three generations, there developed a powerful colonial anti-Chinese discourse of alien-ness. By the 1880s and 1890s a strong labour movement in the Australasian colonies emerged, backed by a deeply integrated nationalism and racism, summed up in the slogan "Australia for the White Man." This intense race-based nationalism was rhetorically driven by a conflation of Chinese culture with disease, a conflation problematically familiar not only in Australian history but in other contexts too.[4] In the Australian colonies this racialised pollution fear was particularly acute, and constitutive of the nation, for several geopolitical reasons. First, the British (that is, "white") colonies of settlement were located inside the non-white Asia Pacific region. Thus the borders of the colonies, and later the nation, were often considered precarious; mythically subject to an invasion from the Asian north (sometimes Chinese people represented the particular threat, sometimes Japanese, sometimes a generic "Asia").[5] This anxious racial and national geopolitical identity was precisely what drove the (always too strident) idea of White Australia from the 1880s through to the Second World War. Second, the problematically common anti-Chinese sentiment of the late nineteenth century coincided with the self-conscious nation-forming around the federation of the six colonies into the Commonwealth of Australia in 1901. Third, the new nation was also an island continent. Surrounded by oceans, a popular as well as an expert culture developed whereby Australia was understood as pure but vulnerable in both health terms and race terms, vulnerable both to "aliens" and to "their" diseases. In this period, questions of race, disease, and immigration were not just incidental or coincidental to Australian nationalism but fully formative of it.[6] One delegate at the Australasian Sanitary Conference of 1884 put it this way: "it is important to discourage as far as practicable the advent of Chinese population in Australasia, as we are of opinion that from such immigrants leprosy may become established as an endemic disease."[7] Early race-based immigration screening thus began: "in the opinion of this Conference, a special examination should be made of all Indian and Chinese immigrants upon their arrival in Australasia, in order to ascertain the presence or absence of leprosy among them."[8]

There was significant geographical distance between the island continent that was to become Australia and various endemic foci of disease around the globe. This meant that the communicable-disease profile of the population within the continent was very different indeed from that of Britain, Europe, India, or North America. Smallpox was not endemic, for example, and cholera simply never arrived on the continent. Leprosy certainly received major attention, but the morbidity rates were minimal: perhaps five or six new cases each year were documented. Nineteenth- and twentieth-century epidemiologists and public health policy-makers were geographically hyper-aware of the significance of the island status of the continent. The long sea voyage from Europe via India was useful, rendering visible (that is, symptomatic) any diseased passenger. For these reasons, maritime quarantine regulations were held to very rigidly in nineteenth- and twentieth-century Australia and were often more comprehensive than British or most European regulations. As one expert put it during discussions on federation in 1895: "A code of sanitary regulations for Australia ... with federal quarantine, would give the colonies the best chance of still retaining the proud title of the virgin continent."[9]

Strict quarantine was often argued to safeguard the "purity" of the colonies-turned-nation. One manifestation of this was Australia's Immigration Restriction Act, passed in 1901. Using various legal devices, this effectively acted as a Chinese exclusion act, the legislative base of the infamous white Australia policy. But the Immigration Restriction Act also contained public health powers – the "loathsome diseases" clause. Indeed, the Immigration Act worked in concert with the Quarantine Act (1908), jointly nominating many particular diseases as restricted, the initial list being smallpox, plague, cholera, yellow fever, typhus fever, and leprosy. Notably, tuberculosis was not on the pre-First World War list of quarantinable diseases. The racialising of smallpox and leprosy in Australia – that is, the cultural and rhetorical linking with Chineseness – meant that the Quarantine Act was itself understood as a mechanism of white Australia too: it was understood to keep Australia clean and pure, that is "white."

The white Australia policy was well known internationally in the early twentieth century, partly because it was championed so vigilantly by Australian governments and partly because it was the test case for the principle of racial/national discrimination and sovereignty at the peace conference after the First World War.[10] In fact, this kind of exclusionary immigration act was far more ordinary than extraordinary for the period. From the 1880s onwards there were many versions and manifestations of Chinese exclusion acts or restrictive immigration acts in the United States, in Canada, New Zealand, South Africa, Natal, and more, many of which had some kind of health and disease power of exclusion as well. Elsewhere I have suggested links between the earliest wave of these acts and concern about leprosy: the Australian instance is exemplary, rather than unique.[11] For the purposes of this chapter, however, the point is the intense connection between the idea of "coloured aliens" and "alien diseases." The Australian director-general of health, Dr J.H.L. Cumpston, put this all very succinctly, saying that "Quarantine" guaranteed "National Cleanliness," "the whole object of which is the keeping of our continent free from certain deadly diseases at present unknown amongst us. And secondly the strict prohibition against the entrance into our country of certain races of aliens whose uncleanly customs and absolute lack of sanitary conscience form a standing menace to the health of any community amongst which such aliens are found."[12]

TUBERCULOSIS, 1901–48

Australian policy-makers who imagined and created the 1901 white Australia policy, including the Immigration Restriction Act, seamlessly conflated disease with racial otherness. Tuberculosis, however, was entirely outside this equation, for it was simply not problematised as a racialised alien or an invading disease. Rather, in 1901 tuberculosis was a disease endemically disabling white working- and middle-class families in Australia, in the middle years of life. With respect to tuberculosis, Australia was not a virgin continent at all.

Tuberculosis was only just being conceptualised as communicable at the beginning of the twentieth century. An emerging sense of tuberculosis as a dangerous disease *because* it was infectious had several implications. First, this characterisation became one of the rationales for its spatial management in the new sanatoria, both private and public. New kinds of healthy and responsible citizens were to be produced by these institutions.[13] For Indigenous communities in Australia, tuberculosis was certainly a major, if not the major, cause of death, but various manifestations of informal and formal racial segregation meant that the sanatoria were generally not utilised by, or open to, Aboriginal people in the early to mid-twentieth century. Rather, the system of missions and then reserves already worked to keep the Indigenous community and the white community apart, to some degree. Often in this period of Australian history, racial segregation and health segregation dovetailed.[14]

The second significant shift resulting from the "new" infectiousness of tuberculosis in the early twentieth century was that its management became a duty of the state. As a communicable disease, rather than an individual condition, tuberculosis came to be understood within a discourse of "dangerousness," and government responsibilities for population health and containing epidemic disease were mobilised. Within the tri-level system of government of the new Commonwealth of Australia (local, state, and commonwealth, or federal, levels), many health and welfare responsibilities remained with the middle level, with the "states." Deeply linked to questions of economy and labour, government involvement in managing tuberculosis was an important part of burgeoning systems of welfare, largely promoted under new Labour governments. As in Britain and Germany, this involved crucial innovations in health and invalidity insurance schemes and pensions.[15] Third, the reconceptualisation of tuberculosis as a communicable disease in the early twentieth century implicated the new first level of government, the commonwealth, or federal, government, and its powers over migration and entry. Pulmonary tuberculosis was specifically named in the Immigration Act, first in 1912, and in the Quarantine Act in 1917.[16]

In the nineteenth century, the climate of the Australian and New Zealand colonies and the long sea voyage to them had been seen as therapeutic for British consumptives.[17] Many people made the voyage, and even settled, for this reason. With the reimagining of tuberculosis as communicable and with new commonwealth powers over entry into the nation, the twentieth century was characterised by an increasingly intense government effort to keep consumptives *out of* the country. Rather than providing an open air haven for consumptives from the Old World, quarantine and immigration regulations served increasingly to exclude consumptive Britons on the grounds of their infection. British authorities and individuals began to realise this only gradually. For example, the 1919 British Interdepartmental Committee on Tuberculosis received numerous proposals for the settlement of tuberculous former servicemen "in those Dominions in which the climatic conditions are such as to be likely to aid in the cure of the disease." They found, however, that by 1919 not only Australia but also Canada and South Africa had clauses in their various immigration acts specifically prohibiting people with any form of tuberculosis.[18] Indeed, as the interwar decades progressed, tuberculosis prevention became one of the foremost reasons for increasingly complex and thorough health screening of immigrants. At the same time, because the disease was so endemic with the white population already in the country, at this point in the century the immigration screening mechanism for prevention was by no means the main focus of tuberculosis management.

How, then, did this fit with the race-based rationales of the quarantine and immigration regulations discussed above? Quite simply, the early to mid-twentieth-century Australian focus on Britons and their health was precisely a result of the exclusionary acts. Because of the working of the Immigration Act, so-called coloured aliens were barred from entry into the country or were deported: the vast majority of migrants to Australia for the first half of the century were British and white. [19] The "loathsome diseases" clause, written with Chinese and their "alien" disease in mind, in fact was used primarily to screen intending British migrants. Thus, precisely because of the exclusion act, the entire mechanism of health screening was built around monitoring, inspecting, and screening Britons, either at point of departure or at port of entry, or more commonly both. Before x-rays, this mechanism involved varying levels of clinical examination and certification. One confused and concerned British traveller detailed the procedures in place around 1920:

[In England] we must get a certificate from a doctor that we are in good health, any doctor will do so long as we produce the certificate ... Then there are in London two doctors who gaze at us as we go up the gangway onto the ship just before we sail ... We have no care until we anchor ... and are boarded by the doctor. This doctor stands on the deck and every passenger is made to pass slowly in front of him. At first this process strikes us as farcical ... but our respect for it deepens when we find that the doctor has picked out every person we know of on board who has been at all in ill health ... The doctor made us undress and examined us very minutely. He told that I had a "click," whatever that might be, and that I was not to leave the ship till the Customs officers had seen me ... I then learned that I was reported to be suffering from tuberculosis, that I had been made a prohibited immigrant, and that I must go back to England. [20]

Another intending British migrant from Pembrokeshire, managed to arrive in Fremantle, Western Australia, in 1928. He was also diagnosed with tuberculosis and deported, but the case raised a significant amount of controversy: "how [did] this migrant come to be passed by the Medical Officer in England?" The case elicited concern at the highest bureaucratic level. Director-General of Health Cumpston, for example, wrote personally to the man's mother to determine whether or not he had actually been placed in a sanatorium in England, suggesting not only the rarity with which infected people slipped through the immigration/quarantine line (or more likely were picked up) but also the seriousness with which the screening process was taken. His certificate of medical examination itself suggests the prominence of tuberculosis in the migrant-screening processes by 1928. The first question was, "Have you ever been in a Sanatorium or other institution or attended thereat for the treatment of Tuberculosis?"[21]

The health screening of Britons was not undertaken on the basis of racial *difference* (the Immigration Act had "solved" that). Nonetheless, this kind of health screening was still squarely about the ambition of white Australia. Now understood much more in eugenic terms, screening came to be explicitly about purifying white Australia – segregating externally as well as internally those individuals likely to tarnish, in the language of the time, the whiteness of the nation. In the curious interwar conflation of infection and heredity, people with tuberculosis were seen to be undesirable in terms of the "race" (however configured), and in various ways they were discouraged from reproducing.[22] Not only Australian governments but groups like the Racial Hygiene Association of New South Wales saw immigration as a health issue in terms of excluding "tarnished" whites, consumptives among them.[23]

While the distinction between "native-born" and "alien" is usually a strongly "raced" distinction in Australian history, the history of tuberculosis epidemiology shows how this was not always the case. When it came to (white) British migrants, they were sometimes alien too. As we shall see, under visa regulations from the 1990s, country of origin currently situates people as low, medium, high or very high risk, determining the extent of health screening to be undertaken. This rationality of risk groups began to be honed with respect to British migrants in the first half of the century. While in this period white Australians usually identified themselves as thoroughly British, with respect to tuberculosis distinctions were constantly drawn between Australians and others. In some studies, the categories were "Australian," "British-born," and "foreigners."[24] In others, British and foreign were categorised together: the categories would be more strongly put as "Australians" and "non-Australians," the latter meaning those born in "England, Scotland, Ireland, Wales, or Foreign Countries."[25] Throughout the period between 1901 and 1948, then, tuberculosis was certainly problematised in terms of migration and health screening, amongst other things. But the problem population was the intending British migrant, not the coloured alien. The rationale was not the need to protect a pure Australian community from infection but rather the need to minimise what was already a high prevalence. After the Second World War, this story of tuberculosis, migration, race, and health screening began to change.

THE NATIONAL PREVENTION CAMPAIGN, 1948–76

In the immediate postwar years, tuberculosis was squarely a disease of both the white and the Indigenous populations in Australia. As one senator put it at the debate on what was to be the Tuberculosis Act, 1948: "Tuberculosis strikes at men and women in their most virile years – their most productive and reproductive years. It causes far more deaths among women of child-bearing age than are caused by all the risks of pregnancy combined. The incidence of the disease is greatest amongst the young and active with their most useful years in front of them."[26]

From 1948 until 1976 Australian commonwealth and state governments backed a large-scale intensive anti-tuberculosis campaign that radically altered the incidence of the disease in the country. Morbidity fell from 49.5 per 100,000 in 1949 to 9.9 per 100,000 in 1975.[27] The precursors of this successful campaign were innovations in miniature mass radiography undertaken by the Australian Army in the Second World War. As elsewhere, the reduction largely resulted from effective chemotherapies: streptomycin, first used in a 1947 trial, and isoniazid and PAS (para-amino salicylic acid) in 1953; rifampicin was trialled in 1969.[28] But it also resulted from an intensive and large-scale preventive effort, nationally funded and state-implemented, in particular from the program of active case finding. The 1948 Tuberculosis Act (Cth) made MMR screening compulsory for every person over sixteen years and ensured ongoing commonwealth funding for it. Powers were granted to examine any contact. The act also granted an allowance to people suffering from tuberculosis, in order that they might stop working and undergo treatment at any stage of the disease, which made it different from the older pension requirement for "total and permanent incapacity." In administering the distribution of this allowance, Aboriginal people were specifically excluded until 1965.[29] A National Tuberculosis Advisory Council reporting to state and commonwealth ministers of health oversaw this multi-directional campaign: active case finding, a network of chest clinics, national mass chest x-ray surveys (eventually compulsory in all states), and a standardised case register.[30] BCG vaccination of all white school leavers was introduced in the late 1940s, and with varying consistency through the states, and continued until the mid-1980s.[31] Vaccination programs were intermittently introduced into Aboriginal communities – in Western Australia from 1950 and New South Wales from 1951.[32]

Under this scheme of prevention and treatment, migrant screening continued to be a focus, but a minor one. Government records and Cabinet submissions regarding the Tuberculosis Act commonly made no mention of migration and health screening at all.[33] At other moments, migration entered the debate marginally, with respect to the intake of postwar refugees and migrants from Europe. For example, the Anti-Tuberculosis Association of Western Australia managed to drag a series of ministers for immigration into detailed discussions about the minutiae of the screening process in Europe. "If he or she cannot come here with a certificate of freedom from Tuberculosis, then he or she is not a welcome addition to our population. No migrants at all would be better than migrants bringing Tubercular trouble."[34] It is worth noting that this Western Australian group (Fremantle, near Perth, being the first point of contact for ships from Britain and Europe) were as concerned with British migrants, who were not necessarily x-rayed, as they were with "alien migrants and displaced persons."[35] In other words, while the discussion of migration was changing to some extent, problematising Southern and Eastern Europeans, British people were still considered the major high-risk group. In 1965, for example, 6,597 people applying for migration from Britain, or 38 percent of all British applicants, were rejected on "medical and radiological grounds."[36] Epidemiologists and immigration bureaucrats also argued over the categorisation of "migrant" with respect to tuberculosis as a chronic disease. In 1963, for example, the *Medical Journal of Australia*'s editor wrote: "[T]he Department of Immigration does not regard as a 'migrant' anyone who has been in

Australia for 10 years or more. This may well be logical from their point of view ... But from a medical point of view the origin of people must be kept in mind. To neglect it in the present instance is to ignore the natural history of pulmonary tuberculosis and the fact that endogenous reinfection may occur many years after the initial seeding of tuberculosis."[37]

Historically, medico-legal border control often distils all kinds of social divisions and relations, where distinctions are made between categories of people on grounds of social privilege rather than on epidemiological grounds. In the postwar period strange but perhaps unsurprising delineations were made. For example, until 1968 chest x-rays were required of all British migrants whose passages were financially assisted. But any non-assisted (that is full-fare paying) British migrant did not require a chest x-ray.[38] Under a new section of the Quarantine Act, full-fare British migrants had to produce evidence that they were free from tuberculosis before embarking, and airline and shipping companies were required to see that all migrants produced a certificate declaring that they were free from tuberculosis.[39] But there still remained a real discrepancy between what was required of different people. As A.J. Proust of the Commonwealth Department of Health explained it in 1974: "assisted-passage migrants from the United Kingdom ... are required to undergo the full medical and radiological examination. Full-fare British migrants, on the other hand, are required to furnish evidence that in the twelve months before their arrival in Australia they have had a chest x-ray examination which showed no evidence of active tuberculosis ... All applicants from Europe and the Middle East are required to undergo the complete medical and X-ray examination."[40] This was so despite epidemiological argument that incidence amongst full-fare paying British migrants would be least twice that amongst "native born Australians."[41]

The low rate of tuberculosis toward the end of this postwar period encouraged the gradual re-emergence of the discourse of Australia as pure. Sometimes this discourse created a reactionary politics, where the low incidence meant vulnerability and therefore the need for tight border protection: "With the continued influx of potentially tuberculous people into a very vulnerable country where the tuberculosis incidence was now the lowest in the world, Australia would be wise to continue a policy of vigilance, and to consider measures designed to protect its native-born population."[42] At other times, Australian "healthiness" gave rise to a distinct generosity, now rare in Australian public discussion on migration. The editor of *Medical Journal Australia* wrote in 1963, for example: "It is only fair that amongst the newcomers we should take aboard a percentage of tuberculous subjects, and there is good reason to believe that a healthy country such as ours can do this safely."[43] Indeed in 1960 the Commonwealth government accepted a group of refugees from Austria, Germany, and Italy "whose applications have previously been rejected because of Tuberculosis." They were identified as "World Refugee Project Special Tuberculosis Cases."[44]

The postwar change in the nationality of migrants to Australia led to the repeal of the Immigration Act and its replacement with a new Migration Act in 1958. The notorious "dictation test" – the legal device by which "coloured aliens" had been excluded – was abandoned. However, the public health power of the old act remained, and the current Migration Act (1958), its amendments and regulations, contain complicated and ever-changing health criteria. But first in public health significance came tuberculosis. And significantly, while many prohibited diseases and conditions were added to the regulations governing the Quarantine Act in these years, it was tuberculosis alone that remained specified in the statute itself.

The 1950s and 1960s saw marked changes in migration regulations. These decades also saw a rapid decrease in the domestic incidence of tuberculosis, in both the white Australian population and in the British population, which was still by far the dominant source for Australian immigration. Deemed successful by any standard, the internationally renowned Australian National Prevention Campaign ceased at the end of 1976. Its abandonment coincided with the sudden reception of new refugees from Southeast Asia. Again and again in medical and popular commentary, the great gains of the preventive campaign that ran from 1948 to 1976 were presented as threatened by the changing migration patterns. From the late 1970s, the idea of the "alien" and of alien diseases – the (barely) repressed of Australian history – returned.[45]

"RISKING" THE VIRGIN CONTINENT, 1976–2001

From 1975 increasing numbers of Laotions, Cambodians, and Vietnamese sought refuge and/or migration to Australia, many arriving on the northern borders of the nation by boat; as onshore asylum seekers, in Australian public culture they are "the boat people." In 1976–77, 7,135 refugees entered Australia. The following year it was 7,077 and the number remained around 10,000 each year until 1984.[46] Initially, there was nothing like the tight border restrictions or the popular resistance to asylum claimants from Southeast Asia that characterised Australian policy in the early twenty-first century. But the question of tuberculosis arose almost immediately: questions were asked and answered in parliamentary debate, driven by media reports of tuberculosis amongst Vietnamese refugees.[47] The particular threat of multi-drug resistant tuberculosis focussed concern, even though its incidence has been low in Australia.[48]

In the early 1990s the tuberculosis "problem" was intensified in both the media and the medical domains. This was partly created by World Health Organization's (WHO) declaration of a global emergency for the disease and by the U.S. and New York City episodes, which received a great deal of medical attention in Australia. In November 1994 Australia's Public Health Association organized the first national conference on tuberculosis in twenty-five years. The connection between tuberculosis and immigration was compounded by, and coincident with, a new shift in policy to mandatory detention for all onshore refugee claimants (those who arrived "unauthorised" in the country by air or by boat, seeking asylum). Amongst the most rigid in the democratic world, this extremely controversial mandatory detention policy was in place from 1992, and diminished significantly, though not abandoned in 2008: detention was rationalised, amongst other ways, by the need for health screening. [49] Speaking at the debate on the Migration Amendment Bill, for example, one senator invoked the threatened virgin continent idea: "we are sitting in the middle of an area that is rife with TB, and we are taking a large number of migrants from that area."[50]

At one level, the threat of disease has come to stand for the threat of race: the issue of higher tuberculosis morbidity becomes an acceptable and seemingly neutral way either to object to or limit migration, and especially the granting of asylum status. As the world's nations tightened their borders after the terrorist attacks in the United States in 2001, questions about Australian border security were compounded by the so-called Tampa crisis, which also took place in that month: a Swedish ship rescued an overturned boat filled with hundreds of people aiming to seek asylum in Australia.

The Australian government refused entry either to the ship or to the asylum seekers, shunning any international obligation. A host of new measures were rushed through parliament, known as the Border Protection Legislation. The system of detention was reinforced and defended by the Australian government at the end of 2001 with specific reference to disease: a new information paper released in October 2001 announced that the detention centres were places where "former terrorists" might be incarcerated and where "tuberculosis, typhoid and Hansen's Disease" were being diagnosed.[51]

In the last quarter of the twentieth century, then, tuberculosis in Australia became a thoroughly "alien" disease and was often discussed within a discourse both drawn from and similar to that which drove aspects of the white Australia policy. Southeast Asian people have been figured as pathologically suspicious *because of* their race, in the way that Chinese-ness and leprosy were conflated by the dominant culture in the late nineteenth century: immigration, race, and disease have again become rhetorically and culturally figured as a tripartite threat to Australian national and racial "security." Sometimes this characterisation has been astonishingly explicit. For example, Senator Pauline Hanson of the then new right-wing One Nation party summarised the threat of "Asian invasion" in her 1996 maiden speech as "tuberculosis, crime and civil war." Queensland senator Bill O'Chee called up the white Australia legacy in response: "Last century it was believed that Asians were responsible for leprosy. That was false, just as it is false to say that Asians are responsible for tuberculosis ...[If] we are to close our borders to these people, then it also follows that we must close our borders and stop Australians going overseas."[52] But as cultural anthropologist Ghassan Hage has argued in his book *White Nation*, the issue of real concern is less the easily identified maverick racism of Pauline Hanson than the more subtle and careful dynamics driving liberal "multicultural" advocacy and policy: the desire for a white (controlled) nation, he argues, is not limited to "racists."[53]

What needs full admission into this debate is that there were, and are, far higher rates of tuberculosis amongst asylum seekers in detention centres than in the Australian population as a whole or in the population of migrants who are subject to screening before arrival. At one level, Pauline Hanson is correct. A study undertaken in 2000–1 in three Australian detention centres for asylum seekers shows an incidence of active tuberculosis at 157 per 100,000. Of

5,742 adults and 1,258 children tested, 7 people were diagnosed bacteriologically, and 2 radiologically and clinically. This compares to the Australian incidence (in 1998) of 4.93 cases per 100,000.[54] Even allowing for the results of a 1999 study that suggests an over-estimation, with a significant number of false-positive results,[55] the higher incidence amongst asylum seekers requires recognition.

A major question, then, is how the issue of disease, race, and geography *can be* articulated without calling up the discourses of white Australia and the accompanying racialised pollution anxiety that so haunts Australian culture. The difficulty lies in gathering and discussing epidemiological data without re-circulating old and deep ideas about the whiteness of a pure but vulnerable Australia in a "dark and diseased" region. These ideas do reappear, however unwittingly: "It is only by constant vigilance that we can hope to maintain our current state of 'paradise,' as we continue to be surrounded on many sides by countries in which tuberculosis and other communicable diseases are recognized by world authorities as being out of control, and with no useful likelihood of control being achieved by Year 2000."[56] Both articulating and not articulating the issue of tuberculosis and migration have been understood as problematic. For example, in 1992 a Labor MP "called for stricter health screening procedures, which he thought had not been enforced for fears of (the enforcers) being branded racist."[57] Simply denying or reversing the epidemiological connection, as Senator O'Chee did in response to Pauline Hanson, is not a subtle enough response.

In looking for and decoding the racism that lingers in Australian migration policy, or, as Hage puts it, the internal managing of national otherness,[58] one approach is to think critically about which population is problematised, why, and how. More to the point, it is to think about which populations are *not* problematised, either epidemiologically or in terms of screening policy. O'Chee's reversal of the problematised population – suggesting restrictions on Australian's travel – is more useful. There is clearly a higher incidence of tuberculosis in some Southeast Asian countries. The current rigid screening procedures may therefore be justified. Yet left unexamined in this geopolitical and epidemiological picture are the thousands of (entirely traceable) eighteen- to twenty-five-year-old Australians who travel through Southeast Asia each year, with no previous exposure to tuberculosis and usually without BCG. Should they also be routinely screened on or before return?[59] Why is this not considered an option? In a globalised world – and SARS and swine flu excepted – it is often the case that migrants are problematised, while travellers are not.

Since 1992 the regulations for entry into the nation have proliferated in complexity, through ever-refining systems of visas (the classes of visa now runs into the hundreds). As in the late nineteenth century, the "virgin continent" is guarded by extremely strict quarantine procedures (incidentally under the original Quarantine Act of 1908). And as in earlier periods, quarantine and health-screening procedures are constantly working bureaucratically in concert with immigration regulation. There are several axes on which this works: period of stay, class of visa, country of origin. Each visa for entry into Australia has a different health criterion attached to it. For example, a tourist visa (normally) requires no clinical examination (or chest x-ray). A temporary resident visa does. But this can change according to the country from which the intending entrant applies. If in the interwar period risk was crudely determined by categories such as "alien," "British," or "native-born," in the 1990s and currently, each nation is grouped within a risk category: different health criteria apply to applicants from each category. In 2002, low-risk countries were Iceland, Monaco, Norway, San Marino, Sweden, and Australia. Medium-risk included Canada, Germany, New Zealand, the United Kingdom, the united States, and Puerto Rico. High-risk included Algeria, Egypt, Fiji, Lebanon, Saudi Arabia, Spain, Turkey, and the United Arab Emirates. And finally, very high risk included Bangladesh, Chile, China, Hong Kong, Indonesia, Korea, Malaysia, Pakistan, Papua New Guinea, Philippines, Portugal, Russia, Singapore, Sri Lanka, South Africa, Vietnam, and Zimbabwe.[60]

Tuberculosis is the prime element in this system of risk assessment. While there was a flurry of bureaucratic concern about HIV and migration in the mid-1980s, positive status does not automatically mean visa rejection. Positive tuberculosis status does, however. The Procedures Advice Manual for 2002 states, "In Australia HIV/AIDS is *not* regarded as a public health risk and it is *not* on the basis of fears of transmission to members of the public that diagnosis of disease might render someone unable to satisfy health criteria (unlike TB, which *is* a public health risk)."[61] Tuberculosis, then, is the only disease for which a discretionary waiver of the health criteria for any visa cannot be made. The manual for clinicians is quite clear, indeed emphatic: "TB is the only health condition prescribed in migration law as *precluding the grant of a visa ... There are no exceptions.*" WHO's declaration of a global epidemic and emergency "with its epicentre in Asia" authorises this emphasis. The manual also refers non-specifically but tellingly to the "public interest" in tuberculosis: "The subject of TB is one that readily achieves a high profile in public interest and comment, given Australia's achievement as a low risk country."[62]

CONCLUSION

The management of tuberculosis in Australian policy and epidemiology has always problematised the place of origin of the infected person: broadly, whether they were native-born to Australia or came from elsewhere. One of the telling aspects of examining tuberculosis epidemiology historically in a country of migration such as Australia is the changing nomenclature through which "those from elsewhere" were categorised. "Immigrant," "alien," "British," "coloured alien," "foreigner," "outside the Commonwealth," the significant marker has sometimes been nationality, sometimes place of birth, sometimes place of residence, race, or region. And for the hyper-scrutinised British migrant, the crucial distinction for health screening was one's "assisted" or "unassisted" passage, broadly, one's class. At times in the twentieth century, the native- born/immigrant distinction has been the central and crucial question in managing tuberculosis in Australia, while at other moments it has been a secondary or tertiary question, falling short of other issues in the minds of those charged with understanding the disease at population level.

The structures for screening were developed almost entirely with respect to the British consumptive, in the decades when eugenic nationalist rationales governed so much social and health policy. In the last few decades, however, tuberculosis management has been almost exclusively concerned with trajectories of global movement *other than* that between Britain and Australia. Between 1901 and 2001 tuberculosis has shifted from being outside the screening process altogether to being the one disease for which entry into Australia is always denied. Seen another way, and from the viewpoint of the problematically dominant culture in Australia, tuberculosis has moved over the century from being "our" domestic disease to "their" exotic disease. In many ways this aligns with the histories of comparable nations, but not every national history has such a deep and explicit connection between racial exclusion, communicable disease, and medico-legal border control.

NOTES

Research for this chapter was funded by the Australian Research Council and by a jointly awarded grant from the British Academy, the Australian Academy of the Humanities, and the Academy of the Social Sciences in Australia.

1 For the United States see Alexandra Minna Stern, "Buildings, Boundaries and Blood: Medicalization and Nation-Building on the US-Mexico Border, 1910–1930," *Hispanic American Historical Review* 79 (1999): 41–81; Nayan Shah, *Contagious Divides: Epidemics and Race in San Francisco's Chinatown* (Berkeley: University of California Press 2001). For Canada see Renisa Mawani, "'The Island of the Unclean': Race, Colonialism and 'Chinese Leprosy' in British Columbia, 1891–1924," *Journal of Law, Social Justice and Global Development* 1 (2003): 1–21.

2 Alison Bashford, *Imperial Hygiene: A Critical History of Colonialism, Nationalism and Public Health* (London: Palgrave Macmillan 2004).

3 For an analysis of the conflation of race, disease, and Chinese immigration in Australia see Desmond Manderson, "'Disease, Defilement, Depravity": Towards an Aesthetic Analysis of Health; the Case of the Chinese in Nineteenth-Century Australia," in Lara Marks and Michael Worboys (eds.), *Migrants, Minorities and Health: Historical and Contemporary Studies* (London: Routledge 1997), 22–48.

4 Shah, *Contagious Divides;* Mawani, "'The Island of the Unclean.'"

5 For the dominance of this idea within Australian history and culture, see David Walker, *Anxious Nation: Australia and the Rise of Asia, 1850–1939* (St Lucia: University of Queensland Press 1999); David Walker, "Survivalist Anxieties: Australian Responses to Asia, 1890s to the Present," *Australian Historical Studies* 120 (2002): 319–30.

6 For a full discussion of these ideas, see Bashford, *Imperial Hygiene,* chaps. 5 and 6.

7 Dr Bancroft, The Australasian Sanitary Conference of Sydney, *Report* (Sydney: Government Printer 1884), 33.

8 Ibid., 33.

9 Dr K.I. O'Doherty, "Federal Quarantine," *Australasian Association for the Advancement of Science* 6 (1895): 840.

10 Sean Bawley, *The White Peril: Foreign Relations and Asian Immigration to Australasia and North America, 1919–1978* (Kensington: University of New South Wales Press 1995).

11 Bashford, *Imperial Hygiene,* chaps. 4, 6.

12 J.H.L. Cumpston, "Cleanliness," Cumpston Papers, National Library of Australia, MS613 Box 7.

13 Bashford, *Imperial Hygiene,* chap. 3.

14 See Suzanne Saunders, "Isolation: The Development of Leprosy Prophylaxis in Australia," *Aboriginal History* 14 (1990): 168–81; Bashford, *Imperial Hygiene.* Indeed, in the Northern Territory, when the reserve system began to relax even a little in the 1950s and Aboriginal people were permitted less intensely surveilled movement, the idea of a sanatorium specifically for them was mooted as a new way of limiting contact and/or movement. By the 1950s of course, sanatorium treatment for the white population was thoroughly outmoded.

15 For this aspect of tuberculosis management in Australia, see Alison Bashford, "Tuberculosis and Economy: Public Health and Labour in the Early Welfare State," *Health and History* 4 (2002):19–40.

16 These diseases and conditions are summarised and tabled in Alison Bashford and Sarah Howard, "Immigration and Health: Law and Regulation in Australia, 1901–1958," *Health and History* 6 (2004): 97–112. Alison Bashford and Bernadette Power, "Immigration and Health: Law and Regulation in Australia, 1958–2004," *Health and History* 7 (2005): 86–101.

17 Linda Bryder, "'A Health Resort for Consumptives': Tuberculosis and Immigration to New Zealand, 1880–1914", *Medical History* 40 (1996): 453–71; J.M. Powell, "Medical Promotion and the Consumptive Immigrant to Australia," *Geographical Review* 63 (1973): 449–76.

18 Report of the Interdepartmental Committee on Tuberculosis (Sanatoria for Soldiers), London, 1919. Copy in National Archives of Australia, A2487 1919/10664.

19 This was in fact never implemented comprehensively: numbers of Chinese, Indian, and Islander families, sometimes in the country for generations at the time of the new act, remained; other individuals were granted entry and exemption from the act from time to time.

20 "Prohibited Immigrants. By One of Them," typescript in JHL Cumpston Papers, National Library of Australia, MS613 Box 7, c. 1920.

21 This case is recorded in "O'Sullivan J – deportation due to tuberculosis," National Archives of Australia, A1 (A1/15) 1928/3804.

22 In Australia, as in Britain, there was never any legislation that made sterilisation compulsory or health certification for marriage compulsory. There were, however, many attempts to enact such legislation.

23 See Bashford, *Imperial Hygiene*, 153–5.

24 J. Burton Cleland, "The Relative Liability of Australian, British-born and Foreigners," *Medical Journal of Australia*, 15 March 1930, 355–6;

25 Advisory Committee of the Racial Hygiene Association of NSW to Stanley Bruce, 13 January 1928, in Report on Immigration (as affecting Racial Values and Public Health), 1928. National Archives of Australia A458 2154/1.

26 Tuberculosis Bill 1948, Second Reading Speech by Senator N.E. McKenna, National Archives of Australia A1658/1 1182/2/1/PART1.

27 T.C. Boag, "Australia Wins Fight to Control Tuberculosis," *Health*, 3, 26 (1976): 8.

28 A.J. Proust, *The History of Tuberculosis in Australia, New Zealand, and Papua New Guinea* (Canberra: Brolga Press 1991), 187–95.

29 Sue Taffe, "Health, the Law and Racism: The Campaign to Amend the Discriminatory Clauses in the Tuberculosis Act," *Labour History* 76 (1999): 41–58.

30 R.M. Porter and T.C. Boag, *The Australian Tuberculosis Campaign 1948–1976*, The Menzies Foundation, n.d.; Jonathan A. Streeton, "Control and Elimination of Tuberculosis in Australia," *Medical Journal of Australia* 162 (1995): 285.

31 The evidence of increasing infection in the workforce was the rationale for vaccinating at the end of school. Porter and Boag, *The Australian Tuberculosis Campaign*, 71.

32 Ibid., 85–6.

33 See, for example, "Tuberculosis Legislation Policy – Cabinet Submissions and Decisions by Cabinet," National Archives of Australia A1658/1 1182/2/1 PART 1. These documents do not mention migration, but detail "case-finding, medical care and isolation, after-care and rehabilitation and the economic security of tuberculosis patients and their dependents ... case-recording, training of personnel, pilot x-ray plants, epidemiological surveys."

34 A.J. Bishop, Secretary, Anti-Tuberculosis Association of Western Australia to Mr N. Lemon, MHR, 1 August 1947. National Archives of Australia A436/1 1950/5/2814.

35 See, for example, letters between Mr A.H. Bishop, on behalf of the association, and Minister for Immigration Arthur Calwell. A436/1 1950/5/2814.

36 See table 2, *Hansards Parliamentary Debate,* House of Representatives, Commonwealth of Australia, vol. 76, 23 February 1972, 186.

37 Editorial, "Tuberculosis and the Migrant," *Medical Journal of Australia,* 6 April 1963, 519.

38 Minister for Health, House of Representatives, *Parliamentary Debates,* 26 October 1960.

39 "Tuberculosis Precautions with Migrants," *Medical Journal of Australia,* 17 August 1968, 342.

40 A.J. Proust, "The Australian Screening Program for Tuberculosis in Prospective Migrants," *Medical Journal of Australia,* 13 July 1974, 36.

41 L. Goldsmith, "Administrative Aspects of Tuberculosis in Australia, 1945–1954," MA thesis, University of Western Australia, 1958, 100.

42 "A Review of Immigrants with Tuberculosis Treated at the Randwick Chest Hospital," *Medical Journal of Australia,* 10 July 1971, 111.

43 Editorial, "Tuberculosis and the Migrant," 519.

44 Memo from Secretary of Department of Immigration, Canberra, to CMO's in Sydney, Melbourne, Brisbane, and Adelaide, 1960. "Acceptance of Refugees with Tuberculosis – Bonegilla Migrant Reception and Training Centre," National Archives of Australia, A2567/1 1960/96C.

45 See, for example, H.E. Williams and P.D. Phelan, "The Epidemiology, Mortality, and Morbidity of Tuberculosis in Australia, 1850–1994," *Journal of Paediatric and Child Health* 31 (1995): 495–8.

46 Gregory B. Goldstein, "A Review of Refugee Medical Screening in New South Wales," *Medical Journal of Australia,* 5 January 1987, 9.

47 See, for example, debate on 7 October 1975, 6 April 1978 House of Representatives, Commonwealth of Australia. 16 February 1977, Senate.

48 See Raelene Allen, "Whither TB in Australia," *Medical Observer,* 22 July 1994, 54–5.

49 Alison Bashford and Carolyn Strange, "Asylum Seekers and National Histories of Detention," *Australian Journal of Politics and History* 48 (2002): 509–27.

50 Senator Newman, *Hansards Parliamentary Debate,* Commonwealth Senate, 25 May 1992.

51 The Department of Immigration and Multicultural and Indigenous Affairs, "Unauthorised Arrivals: Information Paper," October 2001. www.immi.gov.au/illegals/uad/02.thm#7. See Alison Bashford, "At the

Border: Contagion, Immigration Nation," *Australian Historical Studies* 120 (2002): 344–58.

52 Senator O'Chee, *Hansards Online,* Commonwealth Senate, 30 October 1996, 4751.

53 Ghassan Hage, *White Nation: Fantasies of White Supremacy in a Multicultural Society* (Pluto Press Sydney 1998).

54 Kathleen King and Peter Vodicka, "Screening for Conditions of Public Health Importance in People Arriving in Australia by Boat without Authority," *Medical Journal of Australia* 175 (2001): 600–2. See also G.B. Marks, J. Bai, S.E. Simpson, G.J. Stewart, and E.A. Sullivan, "The Incidence of Tuberculosis in a Cohort of South-East Asian Refugees arriving in Australia, 1984–94," *Respirology* 6 (2001): 71–4.

55 Jun Bai et al., "Specificity of Notification for Tuberculosis among Screened Refugees in NSW," *Australian and New Zealand Journal of Public Health* 23 (1999): 411.

56 Jonathan Streeton, "Paradise Lost? Is There a Case for Immigrant Health Screening?" *Medical Journal of Australia,* 5 January 1987, 3.

57 Hansard's Parliamentary Debate, 5 May 1992.

58 Hage, *White Nation,* 107.

59 Streeton, "Paradise Lost?" 2.

60 Immigration Central Office, *Procedures Advice Manual* 3, Schedule 4 – Public Interest Criteria, section 35, Health Examination Requirement by Country and Period and Stay, 9 December 2002.

61 Immigration Central Office, *Procedures Advice Manual* 3, Schedule 4 – Public Interest Criteria, section 39.1, 9 December 2002. Critical scholarship on public health and discrimination often relies on HIV/AIDS management as the ultimate cautionary tale. See, for example, Nicholas B. King, "Immigration, Race and Geographies of Difference in the Tuberculosis Pandemic," in Matthew Gandy and Alimuddin Zumla (eds.), *The Return of the White Plague: Global Poverty and the "New" Tuberculosis* (London and New York: Verso 2003), 40. But it seems to me that the long history (not just the late-twentieth-century history) of tuberculosis screening and categories of difference provides greater insight into the impact of the social on public health policy.

62 Immigration Central Office, *Procedures Advice Manual* 3, Schedule 4 – Public Interest Criteria, section 97, "Overview to TB Procedures," 9 December 2002. Emphasis in original.

6

Importation, Deprivation, and Susceptibility: Tuberculosis Narratives in Postwar Britain

JOHN WELSHMAN

INTRODUCTION

Tuberculosis is now acknowledged as a global health catastrophe. A third of the world's population are infected with the bacillus, eight million people develop active tuberculosis every year, and some two million die. With co-infection with HIV and the emergence of drug-resistant strains that have led in turn to the adoption of the WHO Directly Observed Therapy, Shortcourse (DOTS) strategy, tuberculosis has "apparently made a resurgence almost everywhere in the world."[1] This includes in sub-Saharan Africa, in the former Soviet Union and Eastern Europe, in South America, and in New York and London. In their study, Matthew Gandy and Alimuddin Zumla argue that the idea that infectious disease had been defeated, prevalent in the 1950s, has been proven to be wrong. With hindsight, it is now clear that public health professionals had too short a time horizon, looked only at people, payed little attention to evolution and ecology, and were over-optimistic about development. Gandy and Zumla's overall argument is that the resurgence of tuberculosis is a telling indictment of the failure of global political and economic institutions to improve the lives of ordinary people.[2]

Tuberculosis is directly relevant to recent debates about disease, borders, and geographies of difference. Alison Bashford, for example, has been concerned to integrate the history of health and infectious disease control, arguing they have been part of the legal and technical constitution of "undesirable" entrants. Bashford has argued of Australia that tuberculosis changed from being a disease of civilisation in the early 1900s to, by the 1980s, one associated particularly with migrants, asylum seekers, and refugees. By 2001, it was the only communicable disease nominated in Australian migration regulations.[3] Nick King writes that the resurgence of tuberculosis has led to renewed concern over the borders that separate people and has created a dilemma of how to address inequalities in health while maintaining non-discriminatory policies. Tuberculosis has been a disease associated with immigration, where national and social contexts have been laden with debates about "racial," ethnic, and national difference. Essentialist explanations have explained disease in terms of simple causes and "natural" characteristics, while anti-essentialist approaches have looked at contingent factors. King argues that in general, tuberculosis has served to focus attention on the bodies of people crossing international frontiers and that attention has been diverted from socio-economic and structural problems. He concludes that geographies of difference need to be rethought.[4]

Anne Hardy has shown how perceptions of the character of tuberculosis changed in Britain between 1940 and 1970 following the application of new medical technologies and investigative methods in the diagnosis and tracing of the disease. New techniques such as mass miniature radiography and BCG vaccination meant that the old romanticized image of tuberculosis as a disease of youth was replaced by one centred on children and older people.[5] Nevertheless, while Hardy argues that there was declining interest in the disease, she underplays the specific case of tuberculosis among migrants. It is well known that Britain experienced successive waves of immigration in the postwar period, derived from a combination of "push and pull" factors and both structural and cultural imperatives. From the mid–1950s, researchers began to explore the allegedly higher incidence. While the early papers focused on Irish migrants, the later papers were concerned more with those from India and Pakistan. The location of this research also shifted, reflecting the emergence of large ethnic minority populations in many British cities. While the early research on Irish migrants was based on London, later papers were concerned more with cities such as Birmingham and Bradford and with smaller centres, including Uxbridge and Wellingborough. Chest medicine had low status in the early National Health Service. The interest of researchers in tuberculosis among migrants can be seen in the context of an attempt to revive their specialty.

There has been limited interest in health, "race," and migration in postwar Britain, certainly compared to the literature on the United States.[6] Earlier work has concentrated on the development of the research literature on tuberculosis and migration, the policy response by central government departments and the British Medical Association (BMA), service delivery in specific cities, and comparisons between the United Kingdom and Australia.[7] This chapter responds to King's analysis by examining how far his framework fits the way the debate on migration, tuberculosis, and "race" played out in Britain in the period from the mid-1950s to the early 1970s. These debates were complicated, but for simplicity the chapter looks at three approaches to explaining tuberculosis among migrants. First, I explore how and why some researchers focused on immigration and argued that migrants were "bringing in" the disease. Second, I examine how other researchers directed attention more to contingent structural and socio-economic factors, including nutrition and overcrowding. Third, I trace essentialist explanations and the influence of "race," arguing that older ideas such as the "virgin soil" theory persisted much longer than has previously been realised and were revived in new ideas of "susceptibility" in the postwar period. In each case, I show how these explanations shaped the policy response on the central issue of medical examinations at the ports of entry.

IMPORTATION, IMMIGRATION, AND MEDICAL EXAMINATION

Nick King has noted that immigration has often been identified as the "cause" of tuberculosis. However, while focusing on borders has been politically useful, it has also led to the scapegoating of migrants for social problems. Moreover, he points out that blaming immigration for tuberculosis obscures complexities in the dynamics of the transmission of tuberculosis between individuals and populations. King writes that "focusing too closely on immigrants as vectors of disease conceals the causal roles played by inadequate health care and social and economic injustice in their destination country."[8] In tracing the historical background to these contemporary concerns, the sociological literature has tended to stress the useful-ness of a "port health" interpretation, where the emphasis was allegedly on the "exotic" nature of infectious diseases; the construc-tion of a pathological view of the migrant; and the prevention of the spread of disease to the "native" population.[9]

In the early 1900s, public health doctors had been concerned with the health of Irish and Jewish migrants, but in general there was much less interest in this field, certainly compared to the inter-est in the United States.[10] When a later generation turned belatedly to health, "race," and migration in the 1950s, they argued that tuberculosis was imported by migrants and that its rising incidence could best be tackled by medical examinations at the ports of entry. One influential survey, led by V.H. Springett and based on the expe-rience of the Birmingham Chest Clinic, confirmed that the inci-dence of tuberculosis among Irish and "Asian" migrants was high. From notifications in 1956 and 1957, it was concluded that the Irish cases of tuberculosis were twice as numerous as might be expected and the "Asian-born" four to six times. In the case of the Irish, it was concluded that they formed a "susceptible" non-infected rural population moving into an infectious urban environ-ment. Given the high incidence of tuberculosis in parts of India and Pakistan, on the other hand, the excess notifications in the "Asian" group were said to be "due more to the migration to this country of individuals already tuberculous than to infection of suscepti-bles after arrival."[11] The recommended measures from this analy-sis were BCG vaccination before departure for Irish migrants and x-ray examinations before entry to Britain for migrants from India and Pakistan.

In an article published in the *Lancet* in 1964, Springett argued that those going from an area of very low incidence to one with a higher incidence would be likely to have primary infections in the new environment. On the other hand, groups moving from an area of high incidence to one with lower levels might include a number of cases of tuberculosis. Springett conceded that the high incidence among migrants was exacerbated by poor living conditions but argued that among "Asian" migrants it was due "mainly to their bringing with them the high rates they would experience in their own country."[12] It was only through procedures such as chest x-rays at entry that there was any prospect of controlling and eradi-cating the disease. But again, concern was mitigated by relief that migrants had little contact with the native population. Springett wrote of Birmingham that "it is in some ways fortunate that the immigrant groups with the higher tuberculosis rates – that is, those from Asia – have in general shown little tendency to integrate fully with other groups resident in the city."[13] He maintained his belief in chest examinations at the ports of entry, which would "protect" those already in Britain and were the only satisfactory method of control.[14] As late as 1971, Springett continued to emphasise the importance of facilities for diagnosis and examination of contacts and appeared to place little stress on prevention through improving housing and working conditions.[15]

Other early studies were concerned with particular occupational groups, such as workers in the catering trade. A study of tuberculosis in Soho, London, published in 1961, was carried out by researchers based at a London hospital chest clinic and mass radiography service, and was based on workers in pubs, restaurants, cafes, and coffee bars. Peter Emerson, Gillian Beath, and John Tomkins found from x-rays of 2,611 employees that there was a much higher incidence of "active" cases of tuberculosis per 1,000 workers compared to the incidence in the general population. Tuberculosis was four times more common, especially among those serving alcohol, preparing food, and working in kitchens, and the "Chinese" (mainly from Hong Kong) had the highest prevalence. Emerson, Beath, and Tomkins argued from cases with past or present tuberculosis that half had the disease before joining the catering trade (those from Hong Kong, Italy, and Ireland), while others joined when they were healthy and then developed it (those from Britain and Cyprus). They recommended that all new entrants to the trade should be x-rayed and tuberculin-tested and that BCG vaccination should be provided where necessary. Emerson, Beath, and Tomkins therefore endorsed the value of routine radiographic examinations, especially for the "Chinese."[16]

Work based on Bradford considered the case of arrivals from Pakistan. Here D.K. Stevenson, a consultant chest physician, noted that "Asians" with tuberculosis were first seen at the local chest clinic in 1954 and that by 1961 many of the new notified cases of tuberculosis were from this ethnic group. Estimating that the Pakistani population of Bradford was around seven thousand Stevenson calculated the annual rate of incidence as 1.8 percent, or thirty times greater than that of the "British" population. Around one in five new patients at the chest clinic were Pakistanis. Stevenson also attempted to assess the usefulness of x-ray examinations at the ports of entry through an analysis of Pakistanis with pulmonary tuberculosis seen at the local Middleton Hospital. He estimated that 64 percent of these cases would have been recalled for investigation after screening and endorsed the recommendation of the BMA that migrants should have x-ray examinations at the ports of entry.[17]

Later work by his colleague Dr William Edgar noted that control measures had included attempts to reduce overcrowding, selective use of mass miniature radiography, and comprehensive tuberculin testing. However, Edgar argued that since most of the migrants were single men, worked in hot, humid conditions, spent their free time together, and had poor diets, the emphasis on the relief of overcrowding was of limited value. He concluded that if migrants continued to arrive without medical examinations, the most elaborate systems after entry could not provide a solution.[18] The annual reports of the medical officer of health (MOH) for Bradford echoed Springett's concern about protecting the native population from the spread of exotic diseases. He noted with relief in 1970 that "no case has yet come to light where a locally born resident acquired tuberculosis from an immigrant."[19] Similarly, it is clear that the health of migrants was interpreted solely in terms of the risk posed by infectious disease. The MOH admitted in 1971 that "the detection, or better, the prevention of tuberculosis occupies perhaps 99 percent of the time devoted, in general, to the health of immigrants."[20]

With hindsight, it can be seen that many of these research studies did not have sufficient data to draw sensible conclusions about the relative influences of importation and social deprivation. Nonetheless, what was more important in terms of the development of health policy was not the scientific accuracy of the conclusions drawn but the judgments made on the basis of available evidence. In particular, much of the research published in the 1960s reflected pressure on the part of the BMA that all migrants should have compulsory chest x-rays at the ports of entry. Contemporary newspapers indicate that there certainly was evidence of a moral panic on the question of migration and tuberculosis. In February 1953, the *Daily Herald* carried the headline "TB Aliens Fill Our Clinics," and in August 1960, "TB Alarms the Hospitals: The Disease People Thought Was Beaten" was the banner in the *News Chronicle*.[21]

Moreover, the perceived need for medical examinations was the subject of consecutive recommendations by the BMA and other pressure groups. In November 1956, for instance, the Association of Municipal Corporations recommended that all migrants to Britain should be medically examined before departure and that those suffering from tuberculosis, mental illness, and deficiency, and other infectious diseases be excluded. Similarly the Standing Tuberculosis Advisory Committee of the Central Health Services Council stated in 1959 that only a system of strict medical control of immigration would be completely effective in preventing the spread of tuberculosis.[22]

Exactly why the BMA took this line and whether it was a question of personalities or professional interests is not clear. Probably it perceived that in the absence of an efficient screening system, general practitioners would be left to pick up the pieces. But the emphasis on medical examinations at the ports of entry must also be seen in terms of their wider symbolic value, the limited (and acknowledged) effectiveness of the measures notwithstanding. The extent to which the BMA colluded with this moral panic in the early 1960s can be seen in leader articles and correspondence in the *British Medical Journal* (*BMJ*). In September 1961, for example, the BMA stated that it viewed with concern the admission of migrants without medical checks and argued that all should have chest x-rays. The BMA's council subsequently passed three resolutions to this effect in December.[23] Similarly, in 1962 a *BMJ* leader article concluded from the recent research evidence that "X-ray examination of the chest on entry to Great Britain would detect infection at its source" – a telling example of King's point that immigration was constructed as the cause of tuberculosis.[24]

The *BMJ* clearly felt that the system announced by the Ministry of Health in January 1965, a system that relied on notifying addresses to local MOHs did not go far enough. Contrasting the United Kingdom and Canada, the journal compared the failure to take action on medical examinations in the early 1960s to the delay in taking up diphtheria immunisation in the 1930s. The BMA set up a small working party to investigate the health "problems" of migrants. Its composition was revealing of the way in which the issue was viewed – chaired by the MOH for Manchester, it included a senior port medical officer, chest physician, and radiologist. The list of diseases to be excluded that was drawn up by the working party –

yaws, leprosy, yellow fever, and dysentery, along with mental disorder, drug addiction, and alcoholism – revealed the stress placed on
the threat to others, rather than the health of the migrant. The
working party's main recommendation was that all migrants should
have medical examinations in their country of origin, with further
examinations and follow-up measures after entry, "in view of the
low natural immunity to disease of many immigrants and the social
conditions under which they live."[25]

The 1962 Commonwealth Immigrants Act gave powers to port
health authorities to require those entering as voucher holders (long-
stay migrants) to submit to a medical examination, including a
chest x-ray. The act stated that refusal of entry could be on grounds
of health, a criminal record, security, or previous deportation. In
the case of health, entry could be refused if it appeared to immigration or medical officers that the settler was "a person suffering from
mental disorder, or that it [was] otherwise undesirable for medical
reasons that he should be admitted."[26] Some measures were taken,
including the setting up in February 1965 of an experimental x-ray
screening system at Heathrow Airport. Furthermore, under the
1968 Commonwealth Immigrants Act the provisions for medical
examinations and chest x-rays were extended to the families and
dependants of long-stay migrants. Whether an x-ray was taken or
not, the name and intended address of the migrant, his family, and
his dependants were forwarded to the MOH in the area where he
was planning to settle. Overall, much of the discussion about tuberculosis and migrants was bound up with concerns with "race,"
immigration, and the maintenance of national boundaries.

There are intriguing parallels here with the early twenty-first-
century debate about screening systems. Professional bodies have
continued to be active in calling for tuberculosis screening. The
British Thoracic Society's Code of Practice recommends that all
immigrants or other entrants from Asia, Africa, South and Central
America, and other countries with an incidence of tuberculosis of
40 per 100,000 population per year should be screened.[27] There are
currently ten Port Health Control Units based at major ports and
airports in the United Kingdom. Since the 1971 Immigration Act,
officials have had the right to refer to "medical inspectors" people
who are seeking to enter the country, and they can take into
account the results of a medical examination when deciding to
admit a passenger. Government proposals announced in February

2005 were to implement existing powers by screening visa applicants for tuberculosis on "high-risk" routes and requiring those
diagnosed to seek treatment before they would be allowed entry to
the United Kingdom.[28] Policy in the United Kingdom has therefore
shifted to pre-entry screening for tuberculosis. The law cannot be
used to remove people once they have arrived, and policies have
been drawn up to exclude before arrival.

"ANTI-ESSENTIALIST" NARRATIVES: SOCIO-ECONOMIC AND OTHER CONTINGENT FACTORS

Thus, current debates about the need for screening systems, the way
in which the Port Health Unit system operates, and the wider political context all have striking resonances with debates in the postwar period. Much of the debate about tuberculosis and "race" in
the postwar period focused on immigration as the cause and on the
necessity of establishing medical examinations at the ports of
entry. Nevertheless Nick King also notes that many public health
researchers have adopted "anti-essentialist" methods of explaining
health disparities, emphasising the contingent and multi-factorial
causes of tuberculosis. Rather than focusing on the tuberculosis
bacillus as the single cause, the anti-essentialist viewpoint argues
that multiple factors – poverty, nutrition, homelessness, residential
overcrowding, drug and alcohol abuse, institutionalisation, and
access to health care – contribute to the spread of infection and the
incidence of active cases. These factors are not natural but are
contingent on social conditions.[29]

In cities such as Liverpool, where the population was predominantly white, discussions of tuberculosis in the 1950–70 period
focused on deprivation in the inner-city areas. The concern about
the disease in older men seems to bear out Hardy's depiction of
debates about the position of tuberculosis in the postwar period,
but in illustrating that the disease remained of major concern, local
evidence also challenges her interpretation.[30] Researchers in cities
that did experience the emergence of large ethnic-minority populations also stressed the role played by structural factors. While the
work conducted by Springett and others based on Birmingham had
largely endorsed the concern with "port health" measures, their
approach was contested by other researchers in the West Midlands.

Some of this work was conducted not by the personnel of chest clinics but by the staff of local health departments, and their focus on epidemiology, housing, and prevention reflected their public health perspective. One survey, carried out in July 1956 by the MOH and the chief public health inspector for West Bromwich, confirmed that West Indian, Indian, and Pakistani migrants lived in overcrowded conditions. Communal living was a financial necessity – language, "custom," and circumstances had brought them together initially, and poverty meant they could not move. The authors suggested that their findings did not support the allegation that migrants arrived in Britain suffering from tuberculosis – instead the results indicated "that they contract the disease readily when they work in heavy industry and live in overcrowded conditions."[31]

Other surveys linked the high incidence of pulmonary tuberculosis among Indian migrants to their having developed the disease after arrival and stressed the need for co-operation between general practitioners, public health departments, factory medical officers, and chest clinics. A study based at the Uxbridge Chest Clinic used evidence of the severity of the disease to argue that of a group of thirty-five Indian sufferers, twelve probably had the disease on entry, two had possibly acquired the disease in Britain, and twenty-one had definitely developed the disease after arrival.[32] In Birmingham, Springett had claimed patients already had tuberculosis on arrival in the country, since the disease was predominantly chronic. However, the type of infection found in Uxbridge suggested that many of the Indian immigrants had acquired tuberculosis in Britain. In fact, this survey was based on very small numbers and was highly flawed, since, as we will see, there is no clinically reliable way of distinguishing between primary, post-primary, and reactivated disease. Nevertheless, the inference drawn by the author was that after arrival, health professionals should combine to provide x-rays, tuberculin testing, and BCG vaccination; that they should offer health education in conjunction with local Indian Workers Associations; and that they should attempt to reduce overcrowding.

Uxbridge is located in the London suburb of Southall, and as the pace of immigration increased, the experience of other provincial towns and cities began to attract attention. In Wolverhampton, for example, a study found from new cases notified in 1960 that there were four times as many among Indian migrants as might have been expected in a similar number of local inhabitants. It claimed that of new cases notified in Wolverhampton since 1954, only 19 percent would have been picked up by chest radiography at the time of entry. It was suggested that the rest had developed the disease in England, even though their housing and living conditions, though poorer than those of the host community, were not much worse than in their countries of origin. The study recommended that all Indians should have x-rays after entry and before being accepted on general practitioner lists and that all adults should have annual check-ups.[33] These findings were supported by those of John Corbett, a general practitioner in Wellingborough, who observed the high incidence of tuberculosis among a small group of Indians who had migrated there from the state of Bombay. He concluded that while climate, working conditions, and poor diet were all factors in the high incidence of tuberculosis, "overcrowded living conditions, with consequent possibilities for infection," were probably the most important cause.[34]

Moreover, even those researchers whose studies had endorsed the emphasis on medical examinations at ports of entry appreciated the links between tuberculosis and socio-economic deprivation. Even though Stevenson, in Bradford, had stressed the value of port health measures, he observed that the migrants from Pakistan worked in the textile trade, the engineering industry, and public transport, and he noted that they lived in the older, central wards of the city, which tended to be overcrowded. He claimed from the in-patient survey of hospital cases that while 40 to 50 percent of the cases would have had an abnormal x-ray picture at the time of immigration, it was probable that at least 50 percent of those eventually developing a pulmonary infection acquired it in Britain. He argued that there were two sides to the issue – it was a question both of "the tuberculous immigrant" and of the "susceptible Pakistani."[35] His colleague Dr William Edgar agreed that the arrivals in Bradford from Pakistan worked in the local textile trade, foundry work, public transport, and unskilled engineering, and he not only advocated the selective use of mass miniature radiography and tuberculin-testing but also supported attempts to reduce overcrowding.[36]

It seems that the complex nature of tuberculosis itself created the space in which these debates about the relative importance of importation and subsequent development of the disease could occur. Recent clinical studies have shown that the influences of importation and social deprivation are very difficult to untangle.

The natural history of the disease (potentially very long incubation periods, subclinical infection that is difficult to identify except through tuberculin testing, and difficulty in distinguishing primary disease from post-primary or reactivated disease) complicates such research.[37]

The emphasis on the role of structural factors in the transmission of tuberculosis shaped the policy response to the question of medical examinations at the ports of entry. Certainly, it is clear that the pressure from the BMA and other groups in its favour met continued resistance from the Ministry of Health and its successor, the Department of Health and Social Security (DHSS), from the mid-1950s to the early 1970s. As early as July 1955, for example, Iain Macleod, minister for health, had stated that tuberculosis among Irish migrants was not sufficiently serious to justify health checks at the ports of entry.[38] The ministry clearly viewed the proposals, first, to x-ray migrants on arrival and, second, to inform MOHs of the health of migrants going their areas, as alternatives. The ministry held this view even though George Godber, then deputy chief medical officer (CMO), had observed migrant workers being processed quickly in Geneva.[39] There is evidence that the Home Office and the Colonial Office opposed the BMA proposals. One civil servant at the ministry observed wryly in October 1962 that "whatever scheme we propose short of their original somewhat unrealistic campaign in favour of x-raying compulsorily every immigrant before he was admitted, is likely to give us a certain amount of trouble with the BMA."[40]

The socio-economic evidence certainly provided convenient support for the scheme that the ministry favoured. The ministry's permanent secretary conceded in March 1962 that Asian migrants living in poor housing conditions had a higher incidence of tuberculosis than the general population. But he noted that "whether the incidence is much higher than it would be among UK natives living in similar social and economic conditions is not certain."[41] While civil servants may have stuck to this line because they opposed medical examinations at the ports of entry, reports by other advisory bodies and individuals showed an awareness of the role of socio-economic deprivation. In 1966, George Godber, the CMO, wrote that "as many Commonwealth immigrants in their first years in this country tend to live in overcrowded conditions and to be among the lower income groups, the risk of spread of the disease is considerable."[42] Furthermore, in 1969 the CMO observed of migrants that "it is not their importation of infection but development of clinical tuberculosis after arrival that is the chief cause of concern."[43]

However, despite the recognition of the importance of socioeconomic conditions, the policy response centred on increased surveillance at the local level. In Bradford, for example, the main elements of local activity were mass miniature radiography surveys in residential areas favoured by migrants; tuberculin testing in workplaces, such as textile mills; surveys of houses in "multi-occupation," in an attempt to relieve overcrowding; and BCG vaccination for children and adults. In the face of the arguments about importation, central government opted for a policy that was still essentially concerned with surveillance but that moved its site from the ports of entry to those local authorities that received large numbers of migrants. As was shown earlier, it was based primarily not on compulsory chest x-rays at the ports of entry but on the system whereby port medical officers forwarded the addresses of recently arrived people to local MOHs in the cities where they were planning to settle. The MOHs were expected to advise them to register with a family doctor and to provide other services for both children and adults, including tuberculin testing and BCG vaccination.[44]

It was clear from national evidence that this system did not operate effectively. Figures for 1967, for example, revealed that while addresses for migrants were sent to local authorities, only two-thirds of migrants were visited by the staff of local public health departments.[45] Health visitors were employed for some of this work, and tracing migrants was laborious and time-consuming, since the addresses given were often incorrect or temporary.[46] Despite this evidence, the principle that migrants were allowed to enter the country as long as they reported to an MOH was reaffirmed in the 1968 Commonwealth Immigrants Act. A range of factors was involved in the adoption of this policy. One was the advantage of relatively open borders to a government concerned about a growing economy in which the demand for labour outstripped supply. A second was the wider political sensitivity of the Labour government to the whole issue of immigration. A third was related to the practical difficulties involved in attempting to x-ray large numbers of people and the linguistic and other administrative problems that doing so would have created. Thus, it may ultimately have been political pragmatism that led to a policy stance on the issue of medical examinations that appeared to reflect an interpretation of tuberculosis that emphasised socio-economic factors in transmission rather than importation.

This is essentially the same system, with the same inadequacies, that exists in the United Kingdom in the first decade of the twenty-first century. A study in Newcastle Upon Tyne in 1997 found that the port of entry form system alone was inadequate in identifying migrants for screening and that the yield of new cases was extremely low.[47] It was claimed that port health units no longer had the resources to deal with large numbers of migrants and asylum seekers, while the then health authorities had insufficient resources to offer comprehensive contact tracing and screening.[48] Others have argued the British Port Health Screening system identifies only 10 to 40 percent of the new entrants known to the Home Office or registering with general practitioners and that it is "both incomplete and random," because only a proportion of new entrants are accessed and referred for screening. The system operates only at international ports with port health units attached and relies on immigration officers identifying certain categories of travellers and referring them to port health units for screening by port health officers. Screening consists of a brief medical examination and a chest x-ray. All new entrants, whether they have been x-rayed or not, are referred to the consultant in communicable disease control in the primary care trust of the district of intended residence for further screening. However, many primary care trusts do not arrange screening for the new entrants referred to them, on the grounds that they do not have the resources or have other priorities.[49] More generally, compulsory screening for tuberculosis is seen as being based on inadequate evidence, and as having practical and ethical problems.[50]

"RACE" AND SUSCEPTIBILITY

The allegedly higher incidence of tuberculosis among migrants was explained in terms of racial "susceptibility." Nick King has written that essentialist explanations assume intrinsic differences between people. Biological, physiological, genetic, or cultural differences are seen as causing certain people to be more or less susceptible to tuberculosis. A group of people disproportionally affected by a disease is identified as the cause or the source of that disease and as a threat to the public's health. In this way, a disease is identified as coming from outside.[51]

The connections observers made between tuberculosis and "race" have been explored by earlier writers on the United States and other countries. Randall Packard has previously shown how these ideas influenced the way that tuberculosis was conceptualised in South Africa. He has argued that South African medical authorities attributed the high incidence of tuberculosis among Africans and their failure to develop resistance to their inherent susceptibility. This explanation has reflected changing political and economic interests in white South African society, but the message has been constant – the experience of Africans with tuberculosis has been different from that of whites because Africans are themselves different.

Packard argues that the history of tuberculosis in South Africa and the West "has been shaped by the changing alignment of political and economic interests within a rapidly expanding capitalist industrial economy."[52] In particular, the view that Africans were inherently susceptible to tuberculosis because of their lack of contact with the disease (prevalent in the period 1913–38) deflected attention away from environmental conditions and undercut calls for environmental reform.[53] The "virgin soil" ideas of Lyle Cummins were represented in the work of the Tuberculosis Research Committee (1925) – "by continuing to stress the African's lack of tubercularization, Cummins blamed the victim and reduced the liability of the mining industry."[54] Packard locates the high tide of physiological explanations in the late 1930s, as there was subsequently a recognition that more direct action was necessary to improve environmental conditions. He argues that the 1940s saw a more environmental model that placed a greater emphasis on the conditions of African life. Even so, the new environmental discourse contained within it the "myth of the healthy reserve" and continued to blame the victim.[55]

The links between tuberculosis and race in Britain have largely been neglected, although there has been some work on constructions of tuberculosis in the colonies in the interwar period. Michael Worboys and Mark Harrison have examined the constructions of "tropical," "primitive," and "colonial" tuberculosis in Africa and India before the Second World War, suggesting that tuberculosis was constructed and acted upon as a "disease of civilisation."[56]

Worboys, again, has examined tuberculosis and race before the Second World War, showing that Cummins's "virgin soil" theory, along with the notion of "primitive tuberculosis," was influential in Britain and its Empire. Cummins moved from an inherited model to one where there was more emphasis on resistance, and he incorporated data on age-specific mortality. Worboys concludes that in the 1940s there was a decline in the idea that susceptibility to tuberculosis might depend on any racial factor and that in any case environmental factors were most important in policy and practical measures.[57]

Nevertheless, debates about tuberculosis, "race," and migration in Britain in the 1950s indicated that these earlier ideas remained influential and were incorporated in new ideas of "susceptibility." One of the first reports on tuberculosis and migrants was produced by Evelyn Hess and Norman Macdonald in 1954, based on their experiences in hospitals in Hertfordshire and North London. They noted a belief that the Irish migrant was particularly "susceptible" to tuberculosis, and this appeared to be supported by statistical evidence. They set out to investigate the epidemiological implications of this "racial or ethnic susceptibility," and reported the results of a study based on 292 patients with pulmonary tuberculosis in five hospitals.[58] Of these, 104 (36 percent) were Irish, 129 (44 percent) were Londoners, and 59 (20 percent) were born in Britain but had Irish parents or grandparents. Hess and Macdonald argued that the proportion of Irish patients was high – at least three times that expected on the basis of the relative numbers at risk – and that most were from rural areas, in the West and South West of Ireland. Hess and Macdonald acknowledged that there was a structural explanation of this higher incidence. Many of the Irish patients lived in lodgings or had no settled abode; and their "environment and social circumstances" suggested they had a lower standard of living than the Londoners. Moreover, interviews with the Irish patients indicated there was little evidence of a family history of tuberculosis among parents and grandparents. On the other hand, there was more evidence of a family history among those born in Britain, but with Irish parents or grandparents.

In attempting to explain these figures, Hess and Macdonald turned to the ideas of Louis Cobbett and Lyle Cummins. As Worboys has shown, Cobbett in the 1920s had attempted to explore whether the resistance of "civilised man" to tuberculosis was "racial" or individual.[59] By the late 1920s, Cummins had modified his theory of "virgin soil" to describe the non-immune status of people living in isolated areas who had escaped contact with the tuberculosis bacillus.[60] Hess and Macdonald argued that the Irish-born patients had much less exposure to human-type bacilli in childhood and adolescence than those who lived in English cities. Some patients "broke down" owing to reactivation of earlier infections, and this was accelerated by the "altered environment" and the "additional strain" of living in the poor districts of a big city.[61] But what was more important was the low level of natural resistance. Therefore, Hess and Macdonald claimed to reject a theory of "racial weakness" in favour of one related to the epidemiological phase. What they emphasised was the importance of the degree of exposure experienced by earlier generations and the epidemiological phase in the tuberculosis cycle reached by the community concerned; together these created the "susceptible country-dweller."[62] Giving examples of migrants arriving in cities such as London, Glasgow, New York, Calcutta, and Cairo, Hess and Macdonald suggested the same basic pattern – "low degree of inherited resistance, high degree of tuberculin-negativity, susceptible age-group, poor standard of living – providing a distressingly suitable human culture medium for the waiting bacillus."[63] Hess and Macdonald argued that there was little evidence to support hereditary susceptibility on a racial basis but that there was some "transmissible" factor that influenced the resistance of later generations.

Hess and Macdonald provide a striking illustration of how a modified version of the "virgin soil" theory persisted in the early 1950s. Ideas about susceptibility were also apparent in research on "Asian" migrants. C.P. Silver and S.J. Steel, based at the London Chest Hospital, argued from chest radiographs of seven patients from India and the West Indies that some migrants "fail to develop the same degree of acquired resistance as the European at the time of primary infection, so that the subsequent clinical picture may present features of both primary and chronic pulmonary tuberculosis simultaneously."[64] In interpreting tuberculosis among migrants in Wolverhampton, the author of one study wrote that when "young people from stocks susceptible to tuberculosis" moved from isolated rural communities in an underdeveloped country to a crowded industrial environment, they suffered an excessive development of tuberculosis, including unusual forms. He noted that "urban dwellers whose earlier equally susceptible neighbours have long since succumbed to infection before reproducing their genetic inheritance now tend to develop much more chronic disease."[65]

Packard has argued of the South African example that the "myth of the healthy reserve" and the tendency to blame the victim became entwined with the language of environmental reform but led to inaction.[66] This point about the "susceptibility" of both Irish or Asian migrants was reiterated where action was most important – at the local level. Dr Andrew Semple, MOH for Liverpool, wrote in 1956 that the city had a special problem in the number of Irish settlers, "many of whom either already have early tuberculosis or have such a low resistance to the disease that they fall easy victims in the overcrowded conditions in which they all too often live."[67] In 1965, the MOH for Bradford wrote that migrants were "more prone" to tuberculosis than the local population and that special efforts had been made to find migrants who were "particularly susceptible" to it.[68] Another line of attack was through research on "the natural history of the disease in the Asian."[69] This was summed up in the statement that Asian migrants were more susceptible to tuberculosis than those from Western Europe, "whose experience of tuberculosis in the last two centuries has resulted in a considerable innate resistance which has been reinforced by tuberculosis control in this country particularly in the last 50 years."[70] One of the tuberculosis specialists in Leicester wrote in 1962 that "the factors responsible for the higher incidence in the immigrants are probably a combination of lower racial resistance, inadequate nutrition and poor living conditions."[71] He attributed the higher incidence of tuberculosis to both racial and structural factors.

Contemporary textbooks provide one way of exploring how these ideas were spread among the public health workforce. One of the most interesting was published in 1969 by J.S. Dodge, senior medical officer in Bradford. Dodge's own background is revealing. Trained at Barts, Dodge spent two years of his National Service in West Africa seconded to the Royal West African Frontier Force and serving in Freetown and northern Nigeria. Later he joined the Colonial Medical Service and the Northern Nigeria Public Service. During his ten years in Nigeria he worked with medical field units, leaving Nigeria in 1966 and taking up his Bradford post in 1967. In terms of tuberculosis control, Dodge argued that one factor was the "innate resistance" of the individual, a quality lacking in races in

Asia and Africa where tuberculosis was a relatively new disease. Arriving migrants might include those suffering from the disease, but they also might be more "susceptible." He wrote that "the immigrant may by virtue of his race be more susceptible to tuberculosis infection than the indigenous population even when he has acquired a degree of resistance either naturally or by BCG infection."[72] More generally, the Dodge textbook suggests that in interpreting issues of health among migrants, some public health doctors relied on frameworks drawn from colonial medicine.

As with the Irish migrants, ideas of "susceptibility" were used to back up the positions that bodies such as the Ministry of Health had adopted. Indeed, the concept of susceptibility was attractive precisely on account of its ambiguity. Because they opposed compulsory medical examinations at the ports of entry, commentators drew on the well-worn theme of the "susceptible" migrant to argue against the idea that migrants were "importing" tuberculosis. In January 1956, for example, the Ministry of Health's parliamentary secretary wrote that the real problem was "the susceptible people who come for the first time in contact with the stresses and risks of town life here rather than those entering the country in an infectious condition."[73] Much later, in 1964, the Standing Medical Advisory Council noted that some cases among migrants could be missed by x-ray examinations at the ports and that other "susceptible groups" might acquire the disease after entry.[74] Overall, associating tuberculosis with racial difference reduced a complex problem to a single cause. The relative importance of genetic, cultural, and socio-economic vulnerabilities remain important questions in explaining ethnic inequalities in health.[75]

CONCLUSION

This chapter has been concerned with exploring three different approaches – essentialist, structural, and "racial" – to explaining the allegedly higher incidence of tuberculosis among migrants in the early postwar period. Historically, it is artificial to separate the explanations, since early researchers drew on all three. The evidence presented here suggests that in the immediate postwar period, debates about tuberculosis in migrant groups remained highly racialised. In the case of Irish migrants, the disease was presented as one of "susceptible" migrants from rural areas who had

had little previous exposure to tuberculosis and who therefore ran the risk of contracting the disease when they moved to English cities. This risk was presented in part as a consequence of over-crowded living conditions that facilitated the spread of infection, inadequate nutrition that lowered resistance, and an interpretation that emphasised the increased stress of living in an unfamiliar urban environment. Although it was suggested that the "racial" factor had been disproved, in fact this analysis can be seen to have incor-porated elements of the older "virgin soil" interpretation. Like Cummins, Hess and Macdonald combined the virgin soil theory with one where socio-cultural conditions shaped the development of acquired and inherited immunity. What is striking is how these ideas persisted into the early postwar period. The idea that the Irish were inherently susceptible to tuberculosis because of their lack of contact with the disease deflected attention away from environmen-tal conditions in English cities. The idea of racial susceptibility ran alongside environmental explanations but ultimately served to reduce the impact of structural arguments.

In the case of the migrants from India and Pakistan, on the other hand, the "problem" was represented as being one of migrants from areas with a high incidence of tuberculosis moving to areas where there was a low incidence. It was more often asserted that migrants had brought the disease with them, rather than contracted it in Britain. This assertion provided crucial support for the BMA's campaign in favour of compulsory chest x-rays at the ports of entry. This interpretation was resisted, to an extent, by other writers, many of them from the public health community. Instead, they stressed the importance of the work environment, housing, and nutrition. Again, ideas of racial weakness co-existed with a struc-tural interpretation where the argument was that the "susceptibil-ity" of migrants to the disease was aggravated by poor diet and overcrowding. Nevertheless, the blame for Asian susceptibility to tuberculosis continued to be placed largely on the victim, and actual attempts to tackle the environmental factors in the disease remained extremely limited. Focusing on surveillance and biomedi-cal factors meant that it was possible to avoid confronting more radical political and environmental change.

This chapter has attempted to show the long shadows that his-torical perspectives throw on contemporary debates. A historical perspective is helpful in explaining how the screening system that exists today was created and in revealing relationships between science, politics, and policy and continuities in essentialist, structural, and "racial" framings of migration and tuberculosis.

NOTES

The original research for this chapter was funded by the Wellcome Trust; more recent support has been given by the British Academy. I would like to acknowledge the comments made by the participants at the original Sheffield conference in March 2002, and at subsequent seminars, at Birmingham Medical School, in November 2003, and at the Liverpool Medical Institute, in February 2004, where later versions were given as papers. I am grateful to Alison Bashford, Tony Gatrell, and Sally Sheard for comments and suggestions.

1 Leopold Blanc and Mukund Uplekar, "The Present Global Burden of Tuberculosis," in Matthew Gandy and Alimuddin Zumla (eds.), *The Return of the White Plague: Global Poverty and the "New" Tuberculosis* (London: Verso 2003), 100.

2 Alimuddin Zumla and Matthew Gandy, "Politics, Science and the 'New' Tuberculosis," in Gandy and Zumla (eds.), *The Return of the White Plague*, 241.

3 Alison Bashford, "At the Border: Contagion, Immigration, Nation," *Australian Historical Studies* 33 (2002): 351–2.

4 Nicholas B. King, "Immigration, Race and Geographies of Difference in the Tuberculosis Pandemic," in Gandy and Zumla (eds.), *The Return of the White Plague*, 39–54.

5 Anne Hardy, "Reframing Disease: Changing Perceptions of Tuberculosis in England and Wales, 1938–70," *Historical Research* 76(2003): 535–56.

6 On the United States see Alan M. Kraut, *Silent Travellers: Germs, Genes and the "Immigrant Menace"* (New York: Basic Books 1994).

7 John Welshman, "Tuberculosis and Ethnicity in England and Wales, 1950–70," *Sociology of Health & Illness* 6 (2000): 858–82; John Welshman and Alison Bashford, "Tuberculosis, Migration, and Medical Examination: Lessons from History," *Journal of Epidemiology and Community Health* 60 (2006): 282–4; John Welshman, "Compulsion, Localism, and Pragmatism: The Micro-Politics of Tuberculosis Screening in the United Kingdom, 1950–65," *Social History of Medicine* 16 (2006): 295–312.

8 King, "Immigration, Race and Geographies of Difference," 44–6, 48.

9 See, for example, Waqar I.U. Ahmad, "Making Black People Sick: 'Race,' Ideology and Health Research," in Waqar I.U. Ahmad (ed.), *"Race" and Health in Contemporary Britain* (Buckingham: Open University Press 1993): 11–33; Chris Smaje, "The Ethnic Patterning of Health: New Directions for Theory and Research," *Sociology of Health & Illness* 18 (1996): 139–71.

10 On children, see, for example, Bernard Harris, "Anti-Alienism, Health and Social Reform in Late Victorian and Edwardian Britain," *Patterns of Prejudice* 31, no. 4 (1997): 3–34.

11 V.H. Springett, J.C.S. Adams, T.B. D'Costa, and M. Hemming, "Tuberculosis in Immigrants in Birmingham, 1956–1957," *British Journal of Preventive and Social Medicine* 12 (1958): 135–40.

12 V.H. Springett, "Tuberculosis in Immigrants: An Analysis of Notification Rates in Birmingham, 1960–62," *Lancet* (1964), 1: 1091–5.

13 Ibid.

14 V.H. Springett, "Tuberculosis," in G.E.W. Wolstenholme and Maeve O'Connor (eds.), *Immigration: Medical and Social Aspects* (London: J & A Churchill 1966): 56–63.

15 V.H. Springett, "Tuberculosis Control in Britain 1945–1970–1995," *Tubercle* 52 (1971): 136–47.

16 Peter A. Emerson, Gillian Beath, and John G. Tomkins, "Tuberculosis in Soho," *British Medical Journal* (1961), 2: 148–52.

17 D.K. Stevenson, "Tuberculosis in Pakistanis in Bradford," *British Medical Journal* (1962), 2: 1382–6.

18 W. Edgar, "Control of Tuberculosis in Pakistani Immigrants," *British Medical Journal* (1964), 2: 1565–8.

19 Bradford Health Committee, *Annual Report of the MOH, 1970* (Bradford: Bradford Corporation 1971), 57.

20 Bradford Health Committee, *Annual Report of the MOH, 1971* (Bradford: Bradford Corporation 1972), 59.

21 National Archives, London (hereafter NA) MH 55/2275: cutting from the *Daily Herald*, 10 February 1953; NA MH/2277: cutting from the *News Chronicle*, 5 August 1960.

22 J.F. Skone, "The Health and Social Welfare of Immigrants in Britain," *Public Health* 76 (1962): 132–48.

23 Editorial, "The Tuberculous Immigrant," *British Medical Journal* (1961), 2: 1624–5.

24 Editorial, "Tuberculosis in Immigrants," *British Medical Journal* (1962), 1: 1397–8.

25 "Report of the BMA Working Party on the Medical Examination of Immigrants," *British Medical Journal* (1965), 2: 1423–4.

26 *British Medical Journal* (1961), 2: 1297.

27 Joint Tuberculosis Committee of the British Thoracic Society, "Control and Prevention of Tuberculosis in the United Kingdom: Code of Practice 2000," *Thorax* 55 (2000): 887–901.

28 HM Government, *Controlling Our Borders: Making Migration Work for Britain: Five Year Strategy for Asylum and Immigration* (Cm 6472) (London: HMSO 2005), 26, para. 52.

29 King, "Immigration, Race and Geographies of Difference," 43.

30 Hardy, "Reframing Disease: Changing Perceptions of Tuberculosis in England and Wales, 1938–70." See, for example, Liverpool Health Committee, *Annual Report of the MOH, 1961* (Liverpool: Liverpool Corporation 1962), 85.

31 J.F. Skone and S. Cayton, "An Inquiry into the Housing, Health, and Welfare of Immigrant Coloured Persons in a Midland County Borough," *Medical Officer* 97 (1957): 121–6.

32 J.T.N. Roe, "Tuberculosis in Indian Immigrants," *Tubercle* 40 (1959): 387–8.

33 J. Aspin, "Tuberculosis among Indian Immigrants to a Midland Industrial Area," *British Medical Journal* (1962), 1: 1386–8.

34 John T. Corbett, "Tuberculosis amongst a Small Group of Indian Immigrants," *Journal of the College of General Practitioners* 4, no. 31 (1961): 332–7.

35 Stevenson, "Tuberculosis in Pakistanis in Bradford," 1385.

36 Edgar, "Control of Tuberculosis in Pakistani Immigrants," 1568.

37 K. Tocque, M.J. Doherty, M.A. Bellis, D.P. Spence, C.S. Williams, and P.D.O. Davies, "Tuberculosis Notifications in England: The Relative Effects of Deprivation and Immigration," *International Journal of Tuberculosis and Lung Disease* 2, no. 3 (1998): 213–18.

38 NA MH 55/2275.

39 NA MH 55/2632: J.E. Pater to Secretary, 26 October 1962; ibid., E. Russell Smith to Secretary, 31 October 1962.

40 NA MH 55/2634: H.N. Roffey to J.E. Pater, 29 March 1963.

41 NA MH 55/2632, Secretary to the Minister, 14 March 1962.

42 Ministry of Health, *On the State of the Public Health, 1969* (London: DHSS 1970), 70.

43 DHSS, *On the State of the Public Health, 1967* (London: DHSS 1968), 54.

44 Ministry of Health, *Annual Report of the Ministry of Health, 1965* (London: HMSO 1966), 27.

45 DHSS, *On the State of the Public Health, 1967* (London: HMSO 1968), 79–80.

46 Liverpool Health Committee, *Annual Report of the MOH, 1965* (Liverpool: Liverpool Corporation 1966), 46. See, for example, Blackburn Health Committee, *Annual Report of the MOH, 1967* (Blackburn: Blackburn Corporation 1968), 11.

47 M. Lavender, "Screening Immigrants for Tuberculosis in Newcastle Upon Tyne," *Journal of Public Health Medicine* 19, no. 3(1997): 320–3.

48 Sally Hargreaves, "System to Detect Tuberculosis in New Arrivals to UK Must be Improved," *British Medical Journal* 320 (2000): 870.

49 C.A. Van den Bosch and J.A. Roberts, "Tuberculosis Screening of New Entrants: How Can It be Made more Effective?" *Journal of Public Health Medicine* 22 (2000): 220–3. See also Helen Hogan, Richard Coker, Alex Gordon, Margie Meltzer, and Hilary Pickles, "Screening of New Entrants for Tuberculosis: Responses to Port Notifications," *Journal of Public Health* 27 (2005): 192–5; Sally Millership and Amelia Cummins, "Identification of Tuberculosis Cases by Port Health Screening in Essex 1997–2003," *Journal of Public Health* 27 (2005): 196–8.

50 Richard Coker, "Compulsory Screening of Immigrants for Tuberculosis and HIV: Is Not Based on Adequate Evidence and Has Practical and Ethical Problems," *British Medical Journal* 328 (2004): 298–300.

51 King, "Immigration, Race and Geographies of Difference," 41.

52 Randall M. Packard, *White Plague, Black Labor: Tuberculosis and the Political Economy of Health and Disease in South Africa* (Pietermaritzburg: University of Natal Press 1989), 5.

53 Ibid., 201.

54 Ibid., 207.

55 Ibid., 210, 235, 241–2.

56 Mark Harrison and Michael Worboys, "A Disease of Civilisation: Tuberculosis in Britain, Africa and India, 1900–39," in Lara Marks and Michael Worboys (eds.), *Migrants, Minorities and Health: Historical and Contemporary Studies* (London: Routledge 1997), 93–124.

57 Michael Worboys, "Tuberculosis and Race in Britain and Its Empire, 1900–50," in Waltraud Ernst and Bernard Harris (eds.), *Race, Science and Medicine, 1700–1960* (London: Routledge 1999), 144–66.

58 Evelyn V. Hess and Norman Macdonald, "Pulmonary Tuberculosis in Irish Immigrants and in Londoners: Comparison of Hospital Patients," *Lancet* (1954), 2: 132–7.

59 S.L. Cobbett, "The Resistance of Civilised Man to Tuberculosis: Is it Racial or Individual in Origin?" *Tubercle* 6 (1925): 577–90.

60 S. Lyle Cummins, "'Virgin Soil' and After: A Working Conception of Tuberculosis in Children, Adolescents and Aborigines," *British Medical Journal* (1929), 2: 39–41; S. Lyle Cummins, *Primitive Tuberculosis* (London: John Bale Medical Publications 1939).

61 Hess and Macdonald, "Pulmonary Tuberculosis in Irish Immigrants and in Londoners," 135.

62 Ibid., 136.

63 Ibid.

64 C.P. Silver and S.J. Steel, "Mediastinal Gland Tuberculosis in Asian and Coloured Immigrants," *Lancet* (1961), 1: 1254–6.

65 Aspin, "Tuberculosis among Indian Immigrants to a Midland Industrial Area," 1387.

66 Packard, *White Plague, Black Labor*, 243.

67 Liverpool Health Committee, *Annual Report of the* MOH, *1956* (Liverpool: Liverpool Corporation 1957), 75.

68 Bradford Health Committee, *Annual Report of the* MOH, *1965* (Bradford: Bradford Corporation 1966), 69.

69 Bradford Health Committee, *Annual Report of the* MOH, *1966* (Bradford: Bradford Corporation 1967), 60.

70 Bradford Health Committee, *Annual Report of the* MOH, *1967* (Bradford: Bradford Corporation 1968), 59.

71 Leicester Health Committee, *Report of the* MOH, *1962* (Leicester: Leicester Corporation 1963), 75.

72 J.S. Dodge, *The Field Worker in Immigrant Health* (London: Staples Press 1969), 138.

73 NA MH 55/2275: P. Hornsby-Smith to E. Burton, MP, 13 January 1956.

74 Standing Medical Advisory Committee, *Tuberculosis: The Changing Epidemiological Pattern and Its Implications* (London: Ministry of Health 1964), 1.

75 See, for example, James Y. Nazroo, "Genetic, Cultural or Socio-Economic Vulnerability? Explaining Ethnic Inequalities in Health," *Sociology of Health & Illness* 20 (1998): 710–30.

7

Before McKeown: Explaining the Decline of Tuberculosis in Britain, 1880-1930

MICHAEL WORBOYS

INTRODUCTION

Since the 1950s, the views of Thomas McKeown on the causes of the decline of mortality from pulmonary tuberculosis (TB)[1] in Britain have become well known and vigorously debated.[2] McKeown's claim that improved nutrition and standards of living were the principal factor in the halving of mortality from the 1830s to the 1900s continues to exercise medical historians, as well as historical demographers and epidemiologists. One reason for this is the corollary of his argument, namely, that the three other factors he identified – medical intervention, public health measures, and changes in the disease – were relatively minor causes in the overall fall.[3] Readers will be relieved to know that this chapter is not another contribution to what has become known as "the McKeown debate." Instead, it explores the views of the generation of British doctors from the 1880s to the 1930s who first recognised and discussed the long-term fall in TB mortality. Interestingly, none emphasized any of McKeown's four determinants.

From the 1840s, when consistent serial data on disease-specific mortality became available, a long-term fall in TB mortality was evident.[4] In 1838 there were 385 deaths per 100,000 living, 205 in 1879, and 133 by 1900.[5] Contemporaries were debating the reasons for the decline as early as the 1880s, and some doctors predicted the extinction of TB in the twentieth century.[6] Such expectations were based not simply on the extrapolation of aggregated data; the same trend was clear in mortality patterns by sex, age, occupation, and region. The rate of decline was similar for males and females, with the gains greatest for those under twenty- five years of age.[7] Moreover, there was hope that technological changes, such as the control of dust levels, would improve conditions in those industries with the worst TB records – mining and metalworking. Also, the "excess" level of TB mortality in urban over rural areas was diminishing, such that there might in the future be an urban rather than a rural mortality advantage.

In analysing contemporary views on the decline of TB mortality, I have identified five groups with distinct explanations. I have termed these groups the insanitationists, the infectionists, the hygienists, the diathesians; and the tubercularisationists. In this chapter, I present each group as a Weberian ideal type around the single factor that they saw as the main determinant of decline. These factors were, in turn, for the insanitationists, general sanitary improvements; for the infectionists, control of person-to-person spread; for the hygienists, hygienic behaviour and lifestyle changes; for the diathesians, elimination of people with inherited susceptibilities; and for the tubercularisationists, the development of acquired, herd immunity. Contemporaries coined two of my labels: the infectionists and diathesians, while the others are my neologisms. For each label it is possible to identify leading spokespersons, though the number and positions of their followers varied. I attempt to link the social position and interests of each group to their ideas, practices, and policies. However, the groups were not exclusive; some doctors supported more than one explanation, often at the same time, while others moved between groups over time. Indeed, the five groups were not contemporaneous; rather, they emerged sequentially and in different contexts, and hence, engagement between them was uneven. The chronology of the emergence and apogee of influence occurred by decade as follows: insanitationists, 1880s; infectionists, 1890s; hygienists, 1900s; diathesians, 1910s; and tubercularisationists, 1920s. There are two important differences between the McKeown debate now and the speculation then: first, all five groups were equally interested in TB morbidity as in mortality; and second, their views were developed in the context of policy as their authors and proponents struggled to shape preventive and control measures. Hence, my discussion, although framed at quite a high level of abstraction, is as much about the politics of TB within and without medicine as with explanations of its historical epidemiology.[8]

INSANITATIONISTS

The first person in Britain to write extensively on the decline of TB was Arthur Ransome, a tuberculosis specialist and public health writer from Manchester.[9] Ransome had successful private and hospital practices in the city and was a leading figure in the Manchester and Salford Sanitary Association. He developed a special interest in chest diseases and particularly TB, publishing widely on the subject.[10] Ransome's key claim about the decline of TB was that it was the result of an "unconscious campaign" of sanitary reform since the 1830s and 1840s. In other words, measures that had been implemented to control epidemic, zymotic diseases had also been effective with endemic TB. Ransome drew a direct parallel with the decline of leprosy in earlier centuries, arguing that the two diseases had similar aetiologies, pathologies, distributions, and modes of dissemination and that leprosy "was banished mainly by general sanitary measures ... [and] [t]hat it was scarcely affected by direct efforts at preventing contagion."[11] Leprosy had died out without leprosaria, so the parallel was obvious: "No attempt at isolation has hitherto been made in this country for the suppression of phthisis [TB]; and yet ... the disease is gradually disappearing."[12]

According to Ransome, the single most important sanitary reform had been soil drainage, a view shared by Richard Thorne Thorne, chief medical officer to the British government between 1892 and 1897.[13] Classical sanitarians, that is, those who followed the original Chadwickian notion of linking filth and disease and who saw improvements to the water supply, sewerage, housing, and ventilation as the keys to controlling epidemic diseases, remained in positions of influence in the medical profession and government in the last quarter of the nineteenth century. Around Queen Victoria's Jubilees in 1887 and 1897, they began to celebrate the success of their program, claiming that homegrown sanitation rather than continental medical laboratory science had produced the greatest gains for health and life expectancy.[14] Thorne Thorne argued that improvements had been made, initially, because of sound epidemiological knowledge and, latterly, because of bacteriological understandings, along with the recognition that different diseases required different solutions.[15] Accordingly, he argued that the decline in the incidence of smallpox was a triumph for vaccination and the rigorous application of legislation. The incidence of typhoid fever and cholera, he said, had been reduced by greater cleanliness and sanitary engineering. Paradoxically, no specific sanitary measures had been taken against TB, yet its decline had been amongst the most remarkable.

Ransome's views were also a synthesis of old and new, linking drainage, ventilation, housing, and temperance with new bacteriological ideas.[16] He was influenced particularly by the work of the French microbiologist André-Victor Cornil, who maintained that the tubercle bacillus was spread, not directly from person to person, but indirectly with an intermediate stage in the environment.[17] In fact, such views were congruent with Max Pettenkofer's "ground water theories" of the spread of epidemic diseases that were much admired by British sanitarians.[18] With TB, Ransome wrote that the phase in the environment was critical, as it was in damp and dark places that bacilli could either remain dormant and/or multiply and/or gain virulence. Thereafter, they would be able to re-infect more people owing to their increased numbers and/or virulence.[19] These features of the bacilli were confirmed in field and laboratory experiments by Ransome, Julius Dreschfeld, and Sheridan Delépine in Manchester around 1890.[20] In this sense, it was literally the condition of the soil – damp earth under and around houses that remained unexposed to sunlight or the drying movement of air – that was the main determinant of the incidence and fatality of TB.

Statistics from post-mortem examinations of city dwellers published in the 1890s showed that most adults were infected with the tubercle bacillus, yet only around ten percent developed symptoms and died of the disease. To explain this pattern Ransome elaborated upon the commonly used seed and soil metaphor for infection, arguing that the physical environment directly affected the virulence and infectiveness of the tubercle bacillus and indirectly affected the bodily constitution and hence the resistance of individuals. Such a model was important in enabling Ransome to justify his view that TB was not particularly infectious: it was not the number of contacts that increased an individual's chances of infection but rather the qualitative aspects of those contacts. Ransome worried about "phthisisophobia" – fear of TB – and how the disease would become more difficult to manage if sufferers hid their condition, were neglected by their families, or were forced onto the streets and into Poor Law infirmaries.[21] He also pointed to differences in occupational mortalities, where the highest rates were

amongst those who worked in public houses and dusty factories –
the most insanitary rather than necessarily overcrowded places. His
overall conclusion was that TB was still best combated by the
"inclusive" measures of sanitary reform rather than the "exclusive," germ-centred approach of the new public health.[22]

Ransome also used epidemiological data to support his case.
First, like Thorne Thorne, he highlighted the fact that the decline in
TB had been steady for over sixty years – the slope on graphs was
almost linear – which, he suggested, pointed to the single, continu-
ous influence of improved sanitation. Second, he referred to the
data that showed the highest mortality rates remained linked to specific occupations and their environmental conditions or to those
areas without developed sanitation, for example, Ireland, where
mortality was rising. Third, he dismissed the claims of the infectionists that notification, isolation, and disinfection had accelerated
the decline, pointing to cities such as Manchester and Sheffield,
which had first introduced such schemes and which showed no
improvement above the average national decline.

Ransome advocated a consistent insanitationist position from the
1880s through to 1915, when he published his collected essays on
TB.[23] From around 1910 he enjoyed support from a new generation
of medical officers of health (MOHs) who emphasised improved
housing and urban conditions as critical factors in reducing the
incidence of TB. In 1912, Edward Hope, the MOH of Liverpool,
wrote on the importance of the "healthy house," a view echoed
in 1915 by Maxwell-Williamson the MOH for Edinburgh.[24] Hope
was advancing the continuing claims of prevention over the new
enthusiasm for treatment in sanatoria – which I will show was
the favoured policy of the hygienists. He cited the effects of slum
clearance and new housing development in Liverpool, which had
reduced overall mortality from 400 per 100,000 to 190 per
100,000 in half a century. Maxwell Williamson maintained that
sanatorium treatment gave only short-term benefits.[25] He argued
that during their stay a patient's health might improve and perhaps
their disease could be arrested but that when they left the open air
and salubrity of the sanatorium, the good work was likely to be
undone by insanitary conditions at home. Thus, the best long-term
solution, which followed from long-run epidemiological trends,
was to improve the sanitary standards of all houses. The implications for policy of the insanitationists was to eschew specific anti-TB

measures and continue to pursue general sanitary improvements, which seemed to infectionists and hygienists an invitation, at best, to use resources inefficiently and at worst to do nothing.[26]

INFECTIONISTS

Infectionists portrayed TB as an urgent problem and pointed to the fact that at the start of the twentieth century, the annual death toll remained above fifty thousand. The leading spokespersons in this group were James Niven, MOH for Manchester, and Arthur Newsholme, MOH for Brighton and then chief medical officer.[27] Followers of the McKeown debate will be aware that Leonard Wilson's attack on McKeown's standard-of-living hypothesis was a reworking of Newsholme's work that claimed the decline in TB resulted from an "unconscious policy" of isolating sufferers in Poor Law infirmaries.[28]

Niven's version of the decline of TB mortality was that sanitary reform had reduced levels of person-to-person infection through improved ventilation, the reduction of overcrowding, the closure of common lodging houses, greater use of disinfection, and, more recently, disease notification, which had allowed specific measures to be targeted at infected individuals.[29] Whereas Ransome focussed on the role of the environment, Niven looked to people and their interactions. Infectionists were clear that policy should be based on the view that "phthisis is simply and plainly an infectious disease ... which may be brought under control by direct public administration."[30] What this meant was reliance on the methods being used to control other infectious and contagious diseases, namely, notification, isolation, and disinfection, and, in the particular case of TB, the tighter regulation of the meat and milk supply. In 1908 Niven maintained that vague ideas about the "human soil" were irrelevant in preventive policies: "If we can intercept the tubercle bacillus, the soil, however receptive, does not, as we have seen, become tuberculous. It thus becomes a question how can we do most good, by improving the individual, by giving him a better environment, or by intercepting the tubercle bacillus before they can assail him."[31] Furthermore, concentrating efforts on the bacillus was the best use of scarce public health resources.

Niven found a valuable and influential ally in Arthur Newsholme, whose large volume *The Prevention of Tuberculosis* was also published in 1908.[32] This volume was an encyclopaedic work that reviewed all aspects of the disease, including the forces that were reducing its incidence. As already noted, Newsholme's version of the decline of TB was that the most important factor had been the isolation of advanced cases. His analysis showed "no constant relation between improved general sanitary circumstances and reduction in tuberculosis," and in a remark clearly aimed at Ransome, he bemoaned those who claimed that "the control of tuberculosis must await the general perfection of sanitary circumstances."[33] That said, he acknowledged the role of many factors in the spread and development of the disease but argued overall that to achieve "the best practical results we must simplify this complexity" – which meant specific measures to halt infection.[34] He concluded that "the diminution of infection outweighs in importance the diminution of the conditions favouring infection."[35]

Other infectionists cited different evidence. For example, in January 1910 Thomas Adam – assistant county medical officer for the West Riding of Yorkshire – presented a paper to the Yorkshire Branch of the Society of Medical Officers of Health on mortality from pulmonary tuberculosis in the county.[36] His analysis of recent registrar-general's returns showed a "remarkable result" in the fortunes of the different ridings of the county (the term "riding" refers to the three administrative sub-divisions of the county). The mainly rural North and East Ridings now had a higher corrected mean annual death rate from TB than the urban, industrial West Riding. Adam concluded that the switch had resulted from the greater resources that urban local authorities enjoyed, which had allowed them to implement specific disease control measures. National epidemiological data had long shown a great "excess" mortality amongst urban males in middle age, which infectionists had linked to the higher exposures of working men at work and play, but these exposures were now much reduced. The low mortality rate amongst women of all ages occurred, of course, because they mostly stayed at home and were not exposed to infection.

However, the infectionists' aim of approaching tuberculosis like other infectious diseases proved problematic. Both the public and the doctors experienced the disease as a chronic condition in adults with a variable prognosis, not as an acute, well-defined infection. In 1910, G.W. Moore, MOH for Huddersfield, argued that the enthusiasm in recent years for notification and putting sufferers in sanatoria had actually been accompanied by a levelling out in the rate of decline of the disease. Revealing his colours as an insanitationist, he surmised that this change had occurred because MOHs had taken their eye off the need to continue to improve general sanitation.[37] In addition, even if isolation was desirable, it seemed impossible to achieve on the necessary scale. The highest incidence of TB was amongst adults, whose long-term segregation was impracticable for local authorities because of the beds and benefits required, and unaffordable for individuals and their family. Indeed, hospitalising advanced cases would have effectively meant providing terminal care for this most insidious of conditions – not an attractive proposition for MOHs, nor something likely to attract funding from local authorities.

HYGIENISTS

A new approach to prevention emerged in the late 1890s and early 1900s in the various national and local anti-tuberculosis campaigns – that of the hygienists.[38] In Britain, the leading figures were elite clinicians, especially those who played a leading role in the National Association for the Prevention of Consumption (NAPC), an organization that targeted three areas: health education, the control of dairies and the meat supply, and the provision of sanatoria.[39] The key message of the hygienists was spelt out by William Broadbent, physician and leading medical statesman, at the foundation of the NAPC in 1898: "If consumption is preventable, it ought to be prevented. If it is curable, it ought to be cured."[40]

The latter claim derived from the evidence cited above that the majority of people who were infected with the tubercle bacillus did not develop TB. Hygienists concluded that the decline in TB had resulted not from fewer people being infected but from an increase in the number of people whose bodies were able to arrest, keep latent, or heal the disease. As Harold Scurfield, the MOH for Sheffield explained in 1911, a key aim of any anti-tuberculosis scheme should be to stop slight disease becoming serious disease.[41] The hygienist's notion of resistance was not the strictly hereditarian one of the diathesians nor the immunologically informed one of the tubercularisationists but one framed in older constitutional terms of physiological vigour, toughness of tissues, and perhaps psychological strength.[42] As one might expect from a group dominated by

clinicians, they saw the decline of TB in terms of the strength of individual bodies, not populations. Thus, they spoke about the "suitability of the soil" and bacilli interfering with the "nutrition" of
cells and causing "inflammation."[43] Hygienists saw a third "unconscious campaign" running through the Victorian era, not the "invisible hand" of sanitary reform, which would have been too slow, nor
greater control of infection by notification and isolation but rather
changes in behaviour and lifestyle. These changes were associated
with greater individual hygienic discipline that made the lungs
tougher and able to arrest the actions of the tubercle bacillus. This
argument comes closest to that of McKeown on the standard of living, but while the hygienists did look to dietary factors, their focus
was on individuals' choices, not socio-economic factors as such.

Many clinicians still thought that there was a hereditary factor in
the "suitability of the soil," so it is unsurprising to find hygienists
speculating on how this had been overcome or compensated for
since the 1830s. Their answer was "healthy living," which was
iconically represented in the new sanatoria: an open-air life that
encouraged deeper breathing and the hardening of the lungs; eating a rich, high-fat diet; abstaining from alcohol, vice, and other
excesses; consuming safe meat and milk; controlling coughing and
expectoration; and enjoying a disciplined, regulated life. Hygienists
looked to voluntary and state institutions to provide sanatoria for
TB sufferers or the cheaper alternative of open shelters at home for
domiciliary treatment. In addition, the NAPC would promote
healthy life styles through their publicity and by lobbying state
agencies to take up the cause.

The hygienists' position and their support of sanatoria was challenged in the mid-1900s. The government commissioned an enquiry
by Herbert Timbrell Bulstrode, who was a medical inspector at the
Local Government Board.[44] His report covered all areas of policy
and practice, but the conclusion that attracted most attention was
that TB had low infectivity and that its decline had resulted from
improvements in general health.[45] Niven, like many MOHs, took
exception to the report's criticism of what it termed the "simple contagion theory" that TB should be approached like any other
infectious disease.[46] Bulstrode drew upon many sources for his
view, but took amongst the most compelling to be the evidence that
TB had not and did not readily spread from patients to the staff of
consumption hospitals. Of course, their staffs were doctors and

nurses who were well educated in the "rules of health" and likely to be disciplined and well-fed individuals.

Sanatoria remained controversial, and one response to the controversy by their supporters was to say that their role was educative as much as curative: they taught patients the "rules of health."[47] Hygienists stressed that individual choices of lifestyle and behaviour had reduced TB mortality, hence, implicitly playing down the role of structural factors such as housing, work conditions, and poverty.[48] Their view was that the individual could and should follow the lessons of history and adopt hygienic behaviours; indeed, it was their duty to their family and the community to do so.

DIATHESIANS

The leading, and perhaps only fully fledged, diathesian before the First World War was Karl Pearson.[49] Now largely known for his eugenic views, he became embroiled in a number of health issues, mostly around the use of statistics in medicine, including the success of sanatorium treatment.[50] However, what is important here are his views on the alleged link between tuberculosis and an inherited factor of susceptibility.[51] As noted already, such views about the vulnerability of individuals with a tubercular constitution were still held by many doctors and were sustained by the clinical experience of the great variability of TB in individuals.[52] Pearson maintained that TB disproportionately struck those who had a specific inherited susceptibility; in fact, these individuals were likely to be the 10 percent of those infected who went on to develop the disease. According to Pearson, the high population densities in cities had produced almost universal infection; hence, natural selection had operated to ensure that those with the susceptibility died, whilst the "insusceptible" survived. Over time, this gave the urban population greater evolutionary fitness. In other words, the "weak" had been and were being selected out of the population, and the "weeding out" was happening at its faster rate in cities. Thus, for Pearson natural selection explained not only the fall in mortality since the 1830s but also the closure of the gap between urban and rural mortalities. In the countryside, many people avoided infection and thus selection pressure; hence, there remained a higher number of healthy, though genetically susceptible, individuals. Pearson saw this as a warning to infectionists (who were working to halt person-to-person spread) and to hygienists (who wanted to treat sufferers and halt the development of the disease) that they were relaxing selection pressures and making things worse in the longer term.[53]

After the First World War, Pearson's views were recast in a new racial context around "virgin soil theory," a concept also used by tubercularisationists.[54] More diathesians emerged, for example, Louis Cobbett, who was university lecturer in bacteriology at Cambridge between 1907 and 1929.[55] In fact, Cobbett was part diathesian and part tubercularisationist, making a distinction between the acclimatisation of an individual to a disease, which he saw as acquired immunity, and the racial inheritance of a group, where immunity was "deeply fixed in the blood of each race."[56] He used the differences in TB mortality amongst immigrant groups in New York who lived in similar environmental conditions as evidence of "a true racial and inheritable capacity."[57] He argued that individual acquired immunity was "superimposed" on the racial type, warning his fellow doctors not to disregard either component. Cobbett's views signalled a growing tendency amongst pathologists from the 1910s to reassert the role of inherited racial factors in susceptibility to TB. Like others, he had been impressed by new evidence from pathological anatomists that showed TB in "civilised races" was chronic and localised in the lungs, whilst in the "primitive and dark races" it tended to be acute and generalised.[58]

These differences had been reported during the First World War in the American armed services and in Asian and African colonial troops brought to the Western Front.[59] In the 1920s, influential post-mortem studies were published by the leading American tuberculosis specialist Eugene Opie on TB in Jamaica, studies that emerged from the interest of American eugenists in racial mixing in the colony.[60] These studies were backed up by more extensive surveys of autopsies in the United States, the majority of which were purported to show that tuberculosis in African Americans tended to affect the lymph nodes and be more disseminated than in whites.[61] It also seemed that the tissues of African Americans lacked the ability to produce fibrous tissue in the lungs.[62] He interpreted this evidence as suggesting that it was not just the immune system that determined responses to tuberculosis but that there were deeper differences that were set in the structure of tissues and organs.

Like eugenists more widely, diathesians shied away from advocating specific measures that would have aided the elimination of those susceptible to TB; instead they counselled against measures that might aid their survival. Bryder and others have shown that diathesian notions were held quite widely amongst the public, being evident in the letters to TB specialists asking for advice about potential marriage partners.[63] For the United States, Wilson has shown the diversity of opinion on TB and heredity even within the eugenics movement, but also how the issue remained alive amongst experts and the public, especially over marriage.[64] The early volumes of the Pearson's journal *Annals of Eugenics* published articles by Percy Stocks on TB in Belfast, though these were as much about continuing Pearson's statistical objections to the results claimed for the sanatorium treatment as they were about TB and heredity.[65]

TUBERCULARISATIONISTS

The leading tubercularisationist in Britain was Lyle Cummins, who, like many doctors who had served in the Empire, transferred his experience and knowledge to the domestic sphere.[66] Cummins had worked in Africa before his appointment as professor of tuberculosis at the Welsh National Medical School in 1912, where he worked until his retirement. Using data collected in the Sudan and Egypt, he published an article in 1912 that argued that TB showed the typical features of "virgin soil" incidence.[67] The term was seemingly first used in relation to reports on the outbreak of measles in the Faroe Islands in 1875, in the context of an absence of acclimatisation to the disease.[68] By the 1900s, the term had been taken up in the context of immunology, where a key factor in determining an individual's susceptibility to infection was prior exposure and opportunities to acquire specific immunities. Cummins termed this process of exposure to TB leading to acquired immunity tubercularisation. He applied the notion to individuals and populations. He assumed that all newborn babies were "virgin soil" and that they acquired immunity to TB through low-level exposure from birth onwards.[69] There was a crucial balance in this process: if infection levels were too high at any age the disease would develop and death was likely to follow. If infection levels were too low, tubercularisation would be ineffective: the individual would not acquire immunity and would remain "open" to TB. The ideal was some optimal level of exposure that allowed the development of immunity but not the disease. With populations, the same processes were writ large, with the most advantageous conditions giving "herd immunity," a term also first used by epidemiologists at this time.[70]

As noted above, Cummins's understanding of this process derived in the first place from the study of colonial populations, not Welsh individuals. Indeed, the conflation of individuals and populations was characteristic of tubercularisationists. Experience in Africa and the evidence of the ways TB was spreading in non-industrialised, rural societies around the world suggested to Cummins that "less civilised" populations were also virgin soil for the bacillus. In some ways, he regarded the tubercularisation of a community as a rite of passage to modernity, analogous to individuals developing immunities on the path to becoming adults. In 1912 he produced a table of the different percentages of positive tuberculin skin tests in different populations which he argued both revealed exposure to the bacillus and could be taken as a proxy for immunity.[71] Cummins argued that European societies, through the exposures of individuals to low levels of infection in increasingly hygienic conditions over the nineteenth century, had acquired immunity in each generation. Indeed, this could be seen as part of their adaptation to modern urban, industrial life. The advantage, though biological, also resulted from socio-cultural conditions and their cumulative effects built up over time, owing to greater knowledge of how to prevent the disease. This pattern explained the continuing decline in TB mortality in Britain and other urban, industrial societies.

Further evidence for Cummins's view came in part from Britain and in part from overseas. Higher TB mortality rates amongst rural populations pointed to tubercularisation having been less effective because of lower population densities and poor hygienic conditions. The absence of protective exposure in childhood seemed evident in the earlier age-specific peak in mortality in rural areas. Cummins pointed to epidemiological evidence that rural migrants to cities showed higher mortalities than those born and brought up in cities.[72] Indeed, he was particularly worried about small-town Wales, where there was neither effective tubercularisation nor freedom from exposure, and it was from these towns that migration was more casual.[73] He argued that it was critical to maintain effective levels of tubercularisation and worried that the declining incidence of the disease would present new dangers. Alexander James spelt this out in 1915:

Thus, suppose we could take a portion of the community and practically isolate them in a part of the country where the conditions of life would be ideal, where living conditions comprised the maximum of sunlight and fresh air, where working conditions comprised the minimum strain and worry, where no diseased man or animal would be allowed to enter, and where water, milk, and food would be all absolutely germ-free.

Well, no doubt those people would be very comfortable and happy, and would be all very pleasing to look at; but if after a few generations we took what would be the progeny of these people, and suddenly planting them in a large town like Edinburgh or Glasgow, not necessarily in the slums, we set them to work in their new neighbourhoods, what would be the result? Almost certainly we should find that these "eugenics" would in a very short time be taking every disease that was going, and some probably that had been extinct, and that as compared with original townsfolk, they would be showing a startlingly high mortality from tubercular disease.[74]

The use of the term "eugenics" here is strictly incorrect, as James is referring to acquired, rather than inherited, immunity, though the confusion is perhaps telling.

The population movements of the First World War offered many new opportunities to explore the epidemiology of TB. In 1920, Cummins published the article "Tuberculosis in Primitive Tribes and Its Bearing on the Tuberculosis of Civilised Communities" in the new *International Journal of Public Health* (*IJPH*). He synthesised his earlier work, with new data from the war and studies of age-related mortality, into a more developed version of his 1912 ideas that he now termed a theory of "active immunity acquired by contact with the bacillus."[75] The publication of this article coincided with a major study on the same topic by an American army surgeon, George E. Bushnell.[76] The question of racial susceptibility had been an issue in the United States from the late nineteenth century, though leading tuberculosis experts, such as Maurice Fishberg, maintained confidently that the disease was not a racial problem.[77] He suggested that any advantage with TB mortality enjoyed by Jews was acquired, principally because of the hygienic practices integral to their culture.

Cummins suggested that the tubercularisation of the population was the inevitable consequence of the spread of modern civilisation, indeed, a marker of advancement.[78] If so, was it sensible to work for the eradication of TB? One answer was to argue that TB in Europe and North America had been a long-run epidemic linked to urbanisation and industrialisation. Thus, the European TB epidemic was not the result of civilisation as such but of "faulty" civilisation, one that ignored the "necessary safeguards" for the effective tubercularisation of individuals and the population.[79] The epidemic nature of the TB had been hidden until Koch's announcement of the bacillus in 1882 and the full realisation that TB was both infectious and survivable with the build up of herd immunity. With this knowledge, in future the disease could be rationally managed by ensuring effective tubercularisation.

The continuing decline of TB in the 1920s and 1930s turned such speculations into pressing policy questions, for if incidence levels became very low, Britain would become "virgin soil" once again. The population as a whole would be vulnerable to immigrants carrying the disease, and individuals would be at risk travelling overseas. One hope here was that the progress of science, and especially immunology, would produce the technical fix of artificial immunity, or put another way, artificial tubercularisation – a goal realised with BCG vaccination.[80] Cummins had mentioned this possibility as early as 1923 in his inaugural lecture at the Welsh School when he said: "[If] Nature is gradually getting rid of tuberculosis by a process of unconscious vaccination, then we should, in our efforts at prevention, give a great deal of attention to defending children and susceptible persons from massive doses, and we should concentrate research on efforts to discover a safe and efficient vaccine."[81] Two years later, the *Lancet* was reporting promising results from Calmette's work in France, which was to counter the modern rearing of "a race which would present a 'virgin soil' to infection later in life."[82]

CONCLUSION

The main aim of this chapter has been to show the variety of explanations for the decline of tuberculosis in Britain that were current before Thomas McKeown's work was published in the early 1950s. It is interesting that none of these views was discussed by McKeown and that only one of his specific factors had currency before 1950. Perhaps this adds weight to the suspicion that his style of "argument by elimination" works best against straw men: after all, who ever suggested that medical intervention had led to the decline in TB or that the bacillus had become less virulent? In the critiques of McKeown, some historians have recognised the work of earlier writers and even aligned with their views. An example is Leonard Wilson's explicit adoption of the infectionist position, while with considerable licence, Szreter's arguments can be seen as a synthesis of infectionist and hygienist views.[83] The one thing common to all five groups before 1950 and to those who have addressed the issue since is that all write of an "unconscious campaign" or an "unconscious policy." The terms are problematic as they impute agency without actors or intentionality when they are in fact referring to unanticipated effects of social, economic, and material changes.

A secondary aim of this chapter has been to show the link between particular explanations of the decline in TB mortality in Britain and the interests of particular groups within medicine. Following the approach of my book *Spreading Germs*, I have demonstrated how the professional experiences, positions, and knowledge of the different groups shaped their ideas. And I have shown, moreover, that the views of all the groups were linked to specific TB control policies and that the debates between them were as much about practical policy as about epidemiological understandings. The groups emerged sequentially, following particular changes in medical knowledge, medical technologies, or social priorities that created new professional roles and opportunities. They did not replace one another sequentially; they interacted, co-existed, and in some cases combined. Their relative support and influence varied over time: for example, there were few insanitationists around by the 1920s, while the infectionists and hygienists remained the most influential in shaping policy until 1950.[84] The tubercularisationists had their greatest influence with regard to the emerging problem of TB in the colonial Empire in the 1930s and 1940s.[85]

McKeown's own position and interests as a pioneer of the "new social medicine" have been identified as key determinants of his analysis of TB's mortality decline.[86] It would be anachronistic to expect any of the five groups identified here to have recognised the modern notion of "standard of living" as a factor. Nonetheless, it is noteworthy that none of the possible historical equivalents, such as dietary factors and poverty, were emphasised by any group. Hygienists stressed the role of diet in prevention as well as in treatment – in building stronger bodies that were better able to resist infection. And they stressed the role of wider hygienic practices, but these were set in the context of behavioural changes, not the structural, socio-economic ones favoured by McKeown. Insanitationists and infectionists looked to housing, but more in terms of the physical conditions of buildings than the socio-economic circumstances of residents. What all this shows, in pre- and post-McKeown debates about the decline in TB mortality, is the historical specificity of epidemiological debates, a finding that should reinforce the need for historians of the topic to be reflexive about the situatedness of their own research and writing.

NOTES

1 My use of the term TB for pulmonary tuberculosis in this chapter is strictly unhistorical. I use the term largely because it is convenient, but I contend that it is justifiable for two reasons. First, although tuberculosis could occur in almost any tissue, the pulmonary disease was by far the most common form, and for the period 1880–1930 most references to tuberculosis were to pulmonary tuberculosis. Second, over the nineteenth century there were two main changes in the medical terminology for pulmonary tuberculosis. The terms "consumption" and "phthisis," which defined the condition by its whole body effects, were replaced from the 1830s by pulmonary tuberculosis, which defined it by the localised pathological changes in the lungs. Both terms persisted in medicine to 1900 and after, but after the 1880s, pulmonary tuberculosis was increasingly replaced by "TB," standing for "tubercle bacillus," which defined the disease by its specific cause. There is debate about how much continuity there was in the underlying disease state across these changes; however, contemporaries were confident that the terms were synonymous, which I take as justification for my use of the anachronistic term of "TB."

2 Thomas McKeown, *The Modern Rise of Population* (London: Blackwell 1977). Also see James Colgrove, "The McKeown Thesis: A Historical Controversy and Its Enduring Legacy," *American Journal of Public Health* 92 (2002): 727; R.P.O. Davies et al., "Historical Declines in Tuberculosis in England and Wales: Improving Social Conditions or

Natural Selection?" *International Journal of Tuberculosis and Lung Disease* 3 (1999): 1051–4.

3 Simon Szreter, "The Importance of Social Intervention in Britain's Mortality Decline c.1850–1914: A Re-interpretation of the Role of Public Health," *Social History of Medicine* 1 (1988): 1–37; Sumit Guha, "The Importance of Social Intervention in England's Mortality Decline: The Evidence Reviewed," *Social History of Medicine* 7 (1994): 89–113.

4 There was some debate about whether deaths from lung diseases had simply "moved" categories as the rates ascribed to "disease of organs of respiration" were rising. Arthur Ransome, a renowned specialist in the disease, wrote in 1896 that "Phthisis is a disease so easily recognised in its later stages that it has probably been reported with a fair degree of accuracy all through the period in question, and sooner or later most of the chronic cases of phthisis would have found their way into the death-roll." When considering the matter in 1899, Sir Hugh Beevor commented that TB was "a disease of very slow course, very common occurrence, and easy of diagnosis if fully developed [hence] is less likely to be wrongly certified than most causes of death." Thus, in my discussion I am following my historical actors and assuming that the data on TB mortality trends throughout the nineteenth century was robust and reliable. Louis Cobbett, *The Causes of Tuberculosis*, (Cambridge: Cambridge University Press 1917), 9–13; Linda Bryder, "'Not always one and the same thing': The Registration of Tuberculosis Deaths in Britain, 1900–1950," *Social History of Medicine* 9 (1996): 253–65.

5 Registrar General of Births, Deaths and Marriages in England, *Forty-second Annual Report*, Parliamentary Papers, 1881 [C.2907] XXVII, 97.

6 Arthur Ransome, "The Etiology and Prevention of Consumption," *Lancet* (1890) i: 690.

7 Hugh Beevor, "The Declension of Phthisis" *Lancet* (1899) i: 1006.

8 My analysis complements Linda Bryder's discussion "Causal Factors in Tuberculosis," in her book *Below the Magic Mountain*, where there is an epidemiological component to her, mostly post-1918, discussion about individual responsibility versus environmental factors in contracting the disease. Linda Bryder, *Below the Magic Mountain: The Social History of Tuberculosis in Twentieth-Century Britain* (Oxford: Clarendon Press 1988), 97–129.

9 K.A. Webb, "Ransome, Arthur (1834–1922)," *Oxford Dictionary of National Biography* (Oxford: Oxford University Press 2004) (http://www.oxforddnb.com/view/article/57129 accessed 10 March 2006).

10 Arthur Ransome, *Campaign against Consumption: A Collection of Papers relating to Tuberculosis* (Cambridge: Cambridge University Press 1915).

11 Arthur Ransome, "Tuberculosis and Leprosy: A Parallel and Prophecy," *Lancet* (1896), ii: 103–4.

12 Ibid. "Phthisis" is the Greek term that translates as "wasting," pointing to the whole-body effects of the disease.

13 Richard Thorne Thorne, *On the Progress of Preventive Medicine during the Victorian Period* (London: Shaw and Sons 1888).

14 Lloyd G. Stevenson, "Science down the Drain: On the Hostility of Certain Sanitarians to Animal Experimentation, Bacteriology and Immunology," *Bulletin of the History of Medicine* 29 (1955): 1–26; Michael Worboys, "British Medicine and Its Past at Queen Victoria's Jubilees and the 1900 Centennial," *Medical History* 45 (2001): 461–82.

15 John V. Pickstone, "Dearth, Dirt and Fever Epidemics: Rewriting the History of British 'Public health,' 1780–1850," in Terence Ranger and Paul Slack (eds.), *Epidemics and Ideas: Essays on the Historical Perception of Pestilence* (Cambridge: Cambridge University Press 1992), 134; Michael Worboys, *Spreading Germs: Disease Theories and Medical Practice in Britain, 1865–1900* (Cambridge: Cambridge University Press 2000).

16 Arthur Ransome, *The Causes and Prevention of Phthisis* (London: Smith, Elder 1890).

17 Journal of the American Medical Association 212 (1970), 1371–2.

18 See Worboys, *Spreading Germs,* 114–17.

19 H. Hérard, V. Cornil, and V. Hanot, *La Phtisie Pulmonaire* (Paris: Félix Alcan 1888).

20 Arthur Ransome, "On Certain Conditions that Modify the Virulence of the Bacillus of Tubercle," *Proceedings of the Royal Society of London* 49 (1890–91): 66–73; Arthur Ransome and S. Delépine, "On the Influence of Certain Natural Agents on the Virulence of the Tubercle-Bacillus," *Proceedings of the Royal Society* 56 (1894): 51–6.

21 Arthur Ransome, "The Consumption Scare," *Medical Chronicle* 2 (1895): 241–9. Also see *Lancet* (1883) ii: 991; (1884) i: 482; *BMJ* (1885) i: 213.

22 Worboys, *Spreading Germs,* 234–47.

23 Arthur Ransome, *Campaign against Consumption.*

24 E.W. Hope, "The Expanding Scope of Sanitary Administration," *Public Health* 26 (1912–13): 37–9.

25 A. Maxwell Williamson, Housing Conditions in the Relation to the Spread of Tuberculosis," *Journal of State Medicine* 22 (1915): 87–8.

26 Arthur Ransome, "The Conditions of Infection by Tubercle," *British Journal of Tuberculosis* 1 (1907): 322–6.

27 Joan Mottram, "Niven, James (1851–1925)," *Oxford Dictionary of National Biography* (Oxford: Oxford University Press 2004) (http://www.oxforddnb.com/view/article/57128, accessed 14 March 2006); John M. Eyler, *Sir Arthur Newsholme and State Medicine, 1885–1935* (Cambridge: Cambridge University Press 1997); John M. Eyler, "Newsholme, Sir Arthur (1857–1943)," *Oxford Dictionary of National Biography* (Oxford: Oxford University Press 2004) (http://www.oxforddnb.com/view/article/35220, accessed 14 March 2006).

28 Leonard G. Wilson, "The Historical Decline of Tuberculosis in Europe and America: Its Causes and Significance," *Journal of the History of Medicine* 45 (1990): 366–96; Linda Bryder, "Comments on 'The Historical Decline of Tuberculosis in Europe and America: Its Causes and Significance,' by Leonard G. Wilson," *Journal of the History of Medicine* 46 (1991): 385–62.

29 James Niven, "The Prevention of Phthisis," *Public Health* 5 (1892–93): 282–4; James Niven, "On the Prevention of Tuberculosis," *Public Health* 8 (1895–96): 231–5.

30 James Niven, "The Communicability of Phthisis," *Public Health* 21 (1908): 52–9 and 101–33, 113.

31 Ibid., 110.

32 Arthur Newsholme, *The Prevention of Tuberculosis* (London: Methuen 1908). For a detailed discussion of Newsholme's work on the epidemiology of TB see Eyler, *Sir Arthur Newsholme*, 165–91.

33 Ibid., 211.

34 Ibid., 205.

35 Newsholme, *The Prevention of Tuberculosis*, 310.

36 T. Adam, "Mortality from Phthisis in Yorkshire," *Public Health* 23 (1909–10): 310–20.

37 S.G. Moore, "Some Observations and Heterodox Views on Tuberculosis," *Public Health* 24 (1910–11): 183.

38 I use the term "hygienist" to refer to the holisitic lifestyle orientation of medical views within this group. I am aware that around 1900 the word "hygiene" was increasingly being used as an alternative to "public health" and that its use here might suggest closer links than I want to the insanitationists and infectionists. However, hygienic treatments were widely prescribed by clinicians for individuals, and it is this sense of the word that I am drawing upon.

39 Bryder, *Below the Magic Mountain*, 15–45.
40 William H. Broadbent, "An Address on the Prevention of Consumption and Other Forms of Tuberculosis," *Lancet* (1898) ii: 1103.
41 Harold Scurfield, "Tuberculosis in the British Isles and Measures for Its Prevention," *Public Health* 25 (1911–12): 322–37, also see Harold Scurfield, "Preventive Measures and the Administrative Control of Tuberculosis," *Public Health* 23 (1909–10): 406–8.
42 Worboys, *Spreading Germs*, 194–203.
43 Broadbent, "An Address on the Prevention of Consumption," 1101.
44 *BMJ* (1911) ii: 315–16.
45 Editorial, "The Degree of Personal Communicability of Pulmonary Tuberculosis," *Lancet* (1908) i: 950–1.
46 Niven, "The Communicability of Tuberculosis," 103–5. On the Bulstrode Report see editorial, "The Control of Consumption," *Public Health* 21 (1908): 51.
47 C.H. Garland and T.D. Lister, "A National School for Consumptives: A Study of the Relation of the Sanatorium to the Problem of the Working-Class Consumptive," *Lancet* (1907) i: 677–81.
48 Ronald C. Macfie, "Sanatoriums for the Poor and the Eradication of Consumption," *Lancet* (1905) i: 958–62.
49 Joanne Woiak, "Pearson, Karl (1857–1936)," *Oxford* Dictionary *of National Biography* (Oxford: Oxford University Press 2004) (http://www.oxforddnb.com/view/article/35442 accessed 14 March 2006).
50 J. Rosser Matthews, *Quantification and the Quest for Medical Certainty* (Princeton, NJ: Princeton University Press 1995); Karl Pearson, *A First Study of the Statistics of Pulmonary Tuberculosis* (London: Dulau 1907); Karl Pearson, "The Check through the Fall in the Phthisis Death-Rate since the Discovery of the Tubercle Bacillus and the Adoption of the Modern Treatment," *Biometrika* 12, (1918–19): 374–6.
51 Karl Pearson, *The Fight against Tuberculosis and the Death-Rate from Phthisis* (London: Dulau 1911); Karl Pearson, *Tuberculosis, Heredity and Environment* (London: Dulau 1912); E.G. Pope, *A Second Study of the Statistics of Pulmonary Tuberculosis: Marital Infection*, edited and revised by Karl Pearson, F.R.S, with an appendix on assortative mating from data reduced by Ethel M. Elderton (London: Drapers' Company Research Memoirs), Studies in National Deterioration, no. 3, 1908.
52 Cobbett, *The Causes of Tuberculosis*, 8–119.
53 For a critique of Pearson by a medical officer of health see Ray J. Ewart, "Some Observations Bearing on Professor Pearson's Researches on Tuberculosis", *Public Health* 26 (1912–13): 8–12.

54 Geoffrey R. Searle, "Eugenics and Class," in Charles Webster (ed.), *Biology, Medicine and Society, 1840–1940* (Cambridge: Cambridge University Press 1981), 217–43; Geoffrey R. Searle, *Eugenics and Politics in Britain, 1900–14* (Leyden: Noordhoff International 1976).

55 Louis Cobbett, "The Resistance of Civilised Man to Tuberculosis: Is It Racial or Individual in Origin?" *Tubercle* 6 (1925): 577–90.

56 Ibid., 590.

57 Ibid., 589.

58 S. Lyle Cummins, "Laboratory Research on Clinical Conceptions of Tuberculosis," *British Medical Journal* (1927) i: 762.

59 A. Borrel, "Pneumonie et tuberculose des noirs," *Annales de l'Institut Pasteur* 34 (1920):105; H.C. Clark, "Observations on Tropical Pathology," *American Journal of Tropical Diseases and Preventive Medicine* 3 (1915): 331.

60 Eugene Opie and E. Joyce Isaacs, "Tuberculosis in Jamaica," *American Journal of Hygiene* 12 (1930): 1–61.

61 A. Krause, "Immunity and Allergy in the Pathogenesis of Tuberculosis," *Tubercle* 10 (1928): 22–9.

62 Max Pinner and Joseph A. Kasper, "Pathological Peculiarities of Tuberculosis in the American Negro," *American Review of Tuberculosis* 24 (1932): 463; F.R. Everett, "The Pathological Anatomy of Pulmonary Tuberculosis in the American Negro and in the White Race," *American Review of Tuberculosis* 27 (1933): 411.

63 Bryder, *Below the Magic Mountain*, 221–2.

64 Philip K. Wilson, "Confronting 'Hereditary' Disease: Eugenic Attempts to Eliminate Tuberculosis in Progressive Era America," *Journal of Medical Humanities* 27 (2006): 19–37.

65 P. Stocks and M.N. Keen, *Annals of Eugenics* 1 (1926): 407; P. Stocks, "The Inheritance Factor in Tuberculosis," *Annals of Eugenics* 2 (1927):41.

66 *Lancet* (1949) i: 983.

67 S. Lyle Cummins, "Primitive Tribes and Tuberculosis," *Transactions of the Royal Society for Tropical Medicine and Hygiene* 5 (1912): 245–55.

68 *Lancet* (1875) i: 865–7.

69 Edward L. Collis, "Tuberculosis: Infection, Immunisation, Sensitisation," *Public Health* 35 (1921–22): 113–25.

70 S.F. Dudley, "Some Fundamental Factors Concerned in the Spread of Infectious Disease," *Lancet* (1924) i: 1141–6.

71 L. S. Cummins, "Primitive Tribes and Tuberculosis," *Transactions of the Society of Tropical Medicine and Hygiene* 5 (1912): 248.

72 G.R. Ross, "Types of Tubercle bacilli and the epidemiology of Phthisis," *Lancet* (1925) i: 330–1.

73 S. Lyle Cummins, "Home Infection in Tuberculosis and How to Neutralize Its Dangers," *British Journal of Tuberculosis* 19 (1925): 65–8.

74 A. James, "Public Health and Tuberculosis," *Journal of State Medicine* 23 (1915): 122–3.

75 S. Lyle Cummins, "Tuberculosis in Primitive Tribes and Its Bearing on the Tuberculosis of Civilized Communities," *International Journal of Public Health* 1 (1920): 138–71.

76 George E. Bushnell, *A Study in the Epidemiology of Tuberculosis with Especial Reference to Tuberculosis of the Tropics and of the Negro Race* (London: John Bale, Sons & Danielsson 1920).

77 Maurice Fishberg, *Pulmonary Tuberculosis* (Philadelphia: Lea and Febiger 1919), 67. Bushnell's original intention in 1920 had been to write a monograph on tuberculosis in the tropics and amongst the non-whites races, but like Cummins he was struck by the wider significance of his ideas for industrialised countries and all races.

78 Bushnell, "Epidemiology of Tuberculosis," 210.

79 Arthur Lankester, *Tuberculosis in India: Its Prevalence, Causation and Prevention* (London: Butterworth 1920).

80 Linda Bryder, "'We shall not find salvation in inoculation': BCG Vaccination in Scandinavia, Britain and the USA, 1921–1960," *Social Science and Medicine* 49 (1999): 1157–67.

81 S. Lyle Cummins, "Tuberculosis in Wales," *British Medical Journal* (1922) i: 340.

82 "Vaccination against tuberculosis," *Lancet* (1925) i: 616–17.

83 Szreter, "The Importance of Social Intervention," passim.

84 Bryder, *Below the Magic Mountain*, 130–56.

85 Michael Worboys, "Tuberculosis and Race in Britain and Its Empire, 1900–1950," in Waltraud Ernst and Bernard Harris (eds.), *Race, Science and Medicine, 1700–1960* (London: Routledge 1999), 144–66.

86 Dorothy Porter (ed.), *Social Medicine and Medical Sociology in the Twentieth Century* (Amsterdam: Rodopi 1997); S. Ryan Johansson, "Food for Thought: Rhetoric and Reality in Modern Mortality History," *Historical Methods* 27 (1994):101–26; Simon Szreter, "Rethinking McKeown: The Relationship between Public Health and Social Change," *American Journal of Public Health* 92 (2002): 722–5.

8

"The right not to suffer consumption": Health, Welfare Charity, and the Working Class in Spain during the Restoration Period

JORGE MOLERO-MESA

INTRODUCTION

One of the features most frequently mentioned to highlight the social impact of tuberculosis is that it was the main cause of mortality in every industrialised country in the nineteenth century. In Spain, tuberculosis contributed to around 7 percent of the general mortality rate between 1901 and 1930, which resulted in about thirty thousand deaths each year. Some contemporaries claimed that deficiencies in the data collection and analysis meant the actual figure was as high as seventy thousand; indeed, some estimates multiplied the official number of deaths from tuberculosis by ten. However, high mortality was not the only feature that gave the White Plague the epithet "a social disease." Its association with the working class was very direct: 80 percent of tuberculosis cases occurred in workers between the ages of fifteen and thirty-five. This fact was known by hygienists and doctors who, through their epidemiological studies, linked the incidence of tuberculosis to the proletarian way of life. Along with insufficient food, long working days, and living in unhealthy dwellings, they also pointed to alcoholism, immorality, illiteracy, sexual promiscuity, and masturbation as factors in the genesis and spread of the disease. Tuberculosis was portrayed more as a social plague than as a communicable disease. In addition, some doctors speculated that the disease was leading to the progressive degeneration of the population.[1]

The conditions that were assumed to produce high tuberculosis mortalities were set out as early as 1890 in a report published by the Social Reforms Commission (Comisión de Reformas Sociales). The authors maintained that workers' bodies developed "terribly among abject poverty and lack of space," that they lived "in over-crowded and narrow, gloomy houses lacking ventilation in the big towns, and also in filthy, unhealthy shacks in the rural villages" and that "diseases constantly decimate them."[2] The creation of the Social Reforms Commission in 1883 was the starting point of a period characterised by state intervention in social and welfare reforms.[3] The new initiatives had been started by the Conservative Party with the aim of softening the class struggle by improving the living conditions of the most disadvantaged social strata.[4] An essential role in the reforms was given to social medicine, a discipline that emerged in many countries and was generally associated with the "social question."[5] Spanish historians have tended to ignore the problem of social diseases in the early period of welfare reforms, yet the anti-tuberculosis campaign, along with measures to tackle child mortality, venereal diseases, cancer, malaria, typhus, alcoholism, industrial diseases, and accidents, was as important in Spain as in other European countries.[6] This chapter's starting point is that social medicine's intended pacifying strategy, along with a liberal poor-law system, was an important component in the attempt of the middle class to achieve an accommodation with the working class. This accommodation was necessary because the old system of charitable welfare could no longer sustain the co-existence of a "ruling bloc" of the middle class, the aristocracy, and the Church with the more organized and politically aware working classes.

Supporters of the new social medicine drew upon the new forms of knowledge and specialist practices developed in laboratory medicine and the social sciences. They were mobilised with the aim of changing, both materially and socially, the domestic, communal, and working environments of the working class. Amongst the core features of this new discipline were the systematic use of statistics, the adoption of patient medical care as a preventive strategy, a social vision of disease, and a commitment to "improve the race."[7] The link between the social question and social medicine was obvious and direct, but hygienists also appealed to other interests.[8] First, there was a distinct "economic-demographic factor," which aimed to improve "national efficiency" both in the productive and the military fields through the social reproduction of a healthy population. This idea was evident in the studies that evaluated workers' lives economically, in the evolution of the army's exemptions scheme, and in the eugenic ideas that were aired in most health campaigns.[9] Second, in establishing health as a new value system within the working class, greater self-discipline was promoted too.[10]

In the specific case of tuberculosis, even though its origins were routinely said to be social, public health campaigns did not much concentrate on improving workers' insanitary living and working conditions. Instead they aimed at changing the values, the behaviour, and the way of life of the working class, all of which were promoted as the "real" causes of tuberculosis. Because of the focus on bacteriological problems, especially the tubercle bacillus and the ways that individuals could act to prevent its spread, the social and political origins of the disease were increasingly marginalised. Campaigns that instead highlighted personal responsibility, self-help, and blame further undermined a social conceptualisation of the disease. Fear of disease, created and disseminated by posters, was one element of a hegemonic strategy that aimed to lead the working class to internalise new cultural habits, which would also avoid recourse to direct repression. In other words, the people's attachment to old habits – hygienic, social, and perhaps political – would be suppressed by their own will. This strategy can be seen in the so-called "war against spitting," one of the central issues of the anti-tuberculosis campaigns, as well as in the inner life of sanatoria, where re-education following the principles and practice of hygienic living were often enforced through physical repression.[11] Such measures, along with the provision of a free medical-care system, promised the integration of the working class into the new scientific and industrial system. Turning the masses into *homus hygienicus* carried the hope for the reformers that the public would organize their lives around health and principles derived from medicine.[12]

While medico-social reforms in other countries were supported by compulsory health insurance schemes, for example, in Germany in 1883 and in the United Kingdom in 1911, in Spain they developed within a liberal welfare-charity framework. Both the paltry of budgets of provincial and municipal welfare and the state's apathy towards caring for poor patients meant that campaigns against disease relied heavily on private initiatives. [13]

TUBERCULOSIS AND THE WORKERS' STRUGGLE: THE MADRID CASE

All epidemiological studies carried out in Madrid during the Restoration period reported the miserable living conditions and inadequate diets in the poor districts as the cause of the alarmingly high tuberculosis mortality rates.[14] Vicente Alvarez y Rodríguez-Villamil, physician and councillor on Madrid's city council, studied data on the income and spending of an average family (parents and two children) and concluded that labourers did not consume enough calories to "keep a balanced health state." He calculated that they should consume 3,478 calories a day, but with an average wage of 2.75 pesetas per day, the members of a family of four could afford only 2,503 calories each, resulting in a daily deficiency of 975 calories. He argued that this "constant starvation" left the body without any kind of defence, making these people especially vulnerable to tuberculosis.[15] The imbalance between wages and dietary standards and the consequences for the development of tuberculosis were not unknown to Madrid's proletariat, who used such studies to argue for wage increases. An article published in *El Socialista* in 1899 supported its call for a basic wage of 3 pesetas a day on the grounds of research carried out by two Spanish physicians who had earlier calculated that workers needed 1.50–1.75 pesetas a day per person for a balanced diet. The author stated that living on less than this figure was "ruining the species physiologically, creating generations with low vitality and no physical vigour, and horribly increasing the quota of early mortality from tuberculosis, anaemia, scrofula, and the impoverishment of the race."[16]

The political use of medical knowledge was not the sole preserve of socialists, though. Conservative elements in the middle class rejected the need for social reform on similar grounds. They used evidence that emphasised how "popular habits" such as masturbation, promiscuity, and alcoholism contributed to ill health and argued that illiteracy and ignorance meant that the poor could not understand basic sanitary rules. They also argued that the lack of personal savings, which, in turn, showed the lack of long-term thinking amongst these social classes, meant that their families could not support the costs of treatment for chronic illnesses like tuberculosis or the costs of long periods of convalescence. One of the emblematic etiological factors of tuberculosis was alcoholism, which was said to make workers waste their earnings and make them vulnerable to the disease.[17] The conservative politician Romero Robledo told the Spanish Parliament in 1902 that it was untrue that working classes lived in misery. He asked, "How do cafés, taverns, shops, entertainment places – where well-off classes do not go – survive, both in Madrid and in other places, in the industrious Catalonia, only on the excess of wages of the working class? If spare income was saved and not wasted on such pleasures, the proletariat's situation would improve."[18]

Illiteracy and ignorance were also emphasised in the state-sponsored public health campaigns, especially the need to educate the public on the ways in which tuberculosis was transmitted, on its symptoms, and on the consequences of its development in the body. Guerra y Cortés, the physician working for Madrid's municipal charity, argued that ignorance gave the proletariat fatalistic attitudes, which led them to resign themselves to poverty and sickness.[19] He estimated that the illiteracy rate amongst the workers in Madrid was 45 percent, whilst a study of tuberculosis patients between 1911 and 1914 revealed that 14 percent could not read.[20] Again, the medical studies were contested. For example, the workers' group maintained that tuberculosis originated from misery and not the reverse. In 1899, in reply to an article in *El Liberal* that stated that Madrid's working class was not concerned about hygiene, an editorial in *El Socialista* replied:

[The worker puts hygienic principles into practice] when he reduces his working hours and preserves his energy that has been wasted to the detriment of his health ... when he argues against working himself to the bone and prevents two workers from doing the work of three in the same time ... when he claims a weekly day off to have twenty-four hours rest after six consecutive days of work, in order to entertain himself, perform healthy exercise, and live in a purer atmosphere than exists in the workshops ... when he demands regulation of children's

work to overcome their lack of development and, therefore, to
prevent them from becoming weak and dying at an early age ...
when he demands regulation of women's work and regulations
to prevent industrial accidents ... in short, a worker fights
against what opposes the promotion [of hygiene] in the environment where he lives.[21]

The limited ambitions of the social medicine programs provoked
a reaction from socialist and other reformist groups. [22] A clear
example of Madrid working-class resistance to hygienist approaches
was the campaign against the sales tax between 1904 and 1911.[23]
This tax increased the prices of staple items, and its impact on
dietary standards and thus on the development of tuberculosis was
highlighted by the physician Antonio Espina y Capó in his sub-
mission to the extra-parliamentary commission that was formed in
December of 1905 to review the tax. The commission's report in
April of 1906 supported the abolition of the sales tax on economic
grounds but also pointed out the savings the country would make if
mortality from tuberculosis decreased, "as men's lives have very
high value in the market."[24] Among the conclusions was the observation that the tax was a prime reason why workers could not enjoy
"healthy, cheap food" and live in a "clean, lively, sunny home" –
two key requirements for the control of tuberculosis.[25]

One response to such claims in elite medical circles was to empha-
size workers' responsibility for the development of tuberculosis.
For example, Francisco Cortajerena y Aldebó (1835–1919), in his
speech at the third Spanish conference on tuberculosis in San Sebastián in 1912, argued that the "new socialist theories" were responsible for poverty, because one of their chief weapons – strikes –
depleted workers' resources as they turned the "honest, intelligent
worker into a citizen who has to beg in order not to die from starvation."[26] At the same time, they damaged established industries and
prevented investment in new ones, which increased poverty and, in
the long term, the incidence of tuberculosis. He told the conference,
"Bear in mind that the first thing is living and despite many ideals
proclaimed by those who consider themselves the regenerators of
society, if their concern is not citizens' health, humankind will have
little to thank them for."[27]

CHARITY AS DEFIANCE: THE FESTIVAL OF THE FLOWER

The Spanish system of public welfare was organized on three administrative levels: those of the central state, the province, and the municipality. At the same time, private philanthropic initiatives, such as those organized by the Catholic Church, made private welfare charity an important part of the system.[28] At the beginning of the twentieth century, the new social medicine influenced private welfare charity and brought innovations to those centres devoted to caring for the diseased poor.[29] Dispensaries were no longer limited to care and treatment of the needy but expanded their goals towards the prevention and control of social diseases. The knowledge and actions of the new approaches, grounded in large part in laboratory medicine and seemingly politically neutral science, made them an attractive alternative to older welfare charities, even those operated by the Church.[30]

The system of tuberculosis control that developed in most industrialised countries was based on a structure of dispensaries, sanatoria, and specialist hospitals. In Spain, the construction of sanatoria was rejected on grounds of expense, and the dispensary became the focus of action, being chosen because of its lower cost and its potential to reach sufferers in the working-class areas.[31] Tuberculosis dispensaries were developed as welfare charity centres, hand in hand with private associations that were seeking state support and financial subsidies. The most important ones were the Asociación Antituberculosa Española (Spanish Antituberculosis Association), set up in Madrid in 1903 and the Patronato de Cataluña para la Lucha contra la Tuberculosis (Catalonia Foundation for the Fight against Tuberculosis), established in Barcelona one year later. The former was the base of the first state tuberculosis organization – the Comisión Permanente de Lucha contra la Tuberculosis (Permanent Commission for the Fight against Tuberculosis) created in 1906. This commission was supported by the Ladies Foundation, an aristocratic body led by Queens Victoria Eugenia and María Cristina. During its seventeen-year operation, the commission was unable to lead the anti-tuberculosis campaign effectively, not least because it had an official subsidy of only 100,000 pesetas. In 1907, it absorbed the Catalan Foundation, which became another one of many provincial bodies affiliated with the central organization. The commission's aim was to create a system of dispensaries that provided support to sufferers across the country, but it built only three units in Madrid and subsidized others in a few provincial centres.[32] In comparison to what was achieved in other European countries, the record of anti-tuberculosis activities in Spain was weak.

Official inactivity and the weakness of voluntary measures led in 1912 to a group of Madrid doctors, politicians, and aristocratic women to organize the Liga Popular contra la Tuberculosis (Popular League against Tuberculosis). The aim was to arrange an annual street collection by "young women" to provide funds for the creation and maintenance of a sanatorium in Madrid. At the same time, the league aimed to place hygienic posters across the city that gave instructions on how to avoid and combat tuberculosis and to raise the hygienic consciousness of the public.[33] The first Festival of the Flower, or Tuberculosis Day, was celebrated on 3 May 1913 and was reported as a huge success.[34] A total of roughly 114,000 pesetas was collected, more than the annual official budget for anti-tuberculosis measures provided by the Spanish state. There was a similar collection the following June, this time following a Royal Circular Order and with the support of the second Spanish International Conference against tuberculosis.[35] Women in the league's boards were charged with leading and organizing the collecting stations, which were strategically placed across the city, from where "young [collector] women from all social classes" set off, offering people a cloth flower in exchange for a donation.[36]

CHARITY FAILURE: RED FLOWER DAY

As evidenced in Madrid's paper *El Socialista*, the organized working class was unimpressed with the Flower Festival. In response to the first day in 1913, one report stated that socialists "do not want the tuberculosis problem to be left aside until long-term social change solves it." Rather, it asked for the "fathers of collector ladies and donors" to help by "increasing workers' wages, lowering rents, by not selling denatured food products, [and] by giving up their private country houses."[37] The day after the Festival, *El Socialista* described it as a "particular festival of the Cross of May" that had consisted of improvising "some altars along the public way and asking for donations, thereby robbing the poor."[38] Socialists portrayed the festival as a "show" by conservative elements within the middle class and the Church who were principally concerned to preserve social structures and social relations. Advertisements placed by the Church, which used images of the thin bodies of tuberculosis sufferers, were decried as evoking "fake mercy," especially as the disease was said to have been contracted "due to the mean and heartless society of affluent people, which itself is the most feared bacillus of evil."[39]

Thus, it was argued that the seemingly positive image of the Flower Festival concealed "the true ordeal that the deprived are going through," a point that was supported when the organizers rejected the expression of political slogans at the festival and allowed only "charitable feelings and picturesque, artistic customs." The critique was summed up in the following statement: "Almost all magnates and grandees have also adorned their houses with cloth flowers and huge crosses. In the meantime, poor tuberculosis sufferers are not seen anywhere, and Koch's bacillus is still the owner of the lungs of the destitute, and [he] is killing himself laughing at seeing Madrid's crosses and the naïveté of some liberal authors who have been tricked by reaction, playing along with Catholic ladies and the bishop of the diocese."[40] El Socialista concluded that the coalition of Church and Capital had created tuberculosis by marginalizing workers to the outskirts of the cities and by "placing workers, employees, labourers, and city dwellers in dense, overcrowded conditions at all times."[41]

Immediately after the first festival, reports suggested that only seventy thousand pesetas had been collected, and there were complaints about the "miserable" and "mean" responses, especially amongst those most able to give. For the first time, doctors had become the target of such accusations. Critics contrasted the medical doctors' support of tuberculosis charity with their general and specialist practices, which were said to have become "ignobly commercialised ... by men posing as scientists and men pretending to be respectable. We, the people, know both of them and mind our own business: sweeping them all aside, the only medicine which will remove tuberculosis from mankind."[42]

During the following year, El Socialista tracked the impact of the festival. Its sponsors promoted it as a great success, and the income increased to over one hundred thousand pesetas, though this was reduced to eighty thousand when expenses were deducted. Six months later, the Popular League against Tuberculosis had spent hardly any of the donations, which led to further criticisms that it lacked direction and dynamism. One critic wrote, "giving some little money the 3rd of May for tuberculosis sufferers, one received a cloth daisy that was the symbol of merciful heart, but which most heartless exploiters like to hold."[43] During this time, the working-class papers claimed that landlords had continued to rent unhygienic rooms at high prices, that shopkeepers continued to sell adulterated items, and that employers still paid low salaries for long working days. In other words, the conditions that were widely regarded to be "causing" tuberculosis remained largely unchanged.

The socialist press did not miss a chance to attack Tuberculosis Day when, for example, it was found that in Sevilla more than one thousand pesetas in fake coins had been collected.[44] One headline in 1914 stated, "[o]ne year on, not one tuberculosis sufferer has been cured" by the donations.[45] El Socialista portrayed the Festival of the Flower as a sign of class distance and disdain, an insult to the working classes that was "spitting in the face of those in misery."[46] The response of the Socialist Party to the now annual celebration of the Festival of the Flower was to organize Red Flower Day, in 1915, not for health work but to support El Socialista. The first of May was chosen as the day for young female members to carry out the collection, giving a red flower in exchange for contributions to the journal. First suggested in Asturias, the idea was embraced by the journal as a solution to its monetary crisis.[47] Moreover, according to the socialist leader Andrés Saborit, "our Festival on the 1ST of May [would adorn itself] with a touch of beauty, making it more appealing."[48] After a modest start in Asturias and Madrid, Red Flower Day was soon celebrated in several Spanish towns. [49] An article in El Socialista on the eve of 1 May 1917 admitted that "this very pleasant practice had achieved a remarkable income for our dear journal" and encouraged readers for that year with the claim that the "[r]ed flower flourishes, comrades. Its seed is fertile and beautiful. Long live the red flower!"[50] Red Flower Day became a symbol of social transformation not lacking poetic flourishes: "Now we workers and socialists are going to vindicate flowers. And we have chosen red ones, of a bright colour, as bright are our souls and not matt and cold as the ones of the Pharisees we fight against; blood coloured flowers of life, of strength – socialist flowers."[51]

Flowers, insisted one article, just as when they had been thrown in the path of kings, had been desecrated by "vile creatures" that collected money in the name of religion and most recently by those who had used them to help combat the most "terrible scourge of tuberculosis."

Because of socialist pressure, the Popular League's Festival of the Flower was moved in 1915 to 2 June, away from the workers' festival and any conflict with what was said to be their "peculiar" view of the tuberculosis problem. Seemingly in its place, Red Flower Day spread throughout Spain. In 1916, the summary of the collection carried out by working organizations in some places was released and, when added to previous incomes, reached a figure close to seventy-five thousand pesetas. Journalists on *El Socialista* claimed that socialist women, working by sustaining the press, "did more, infinitely more, for the population's health, for mankind's morality and for physical health than those so noisily collecting pesetas for tuberculosis sufferers in the name of some society's doctrines, of some feelings that are constant viruses of tuberculosis corroding the organisms of the poor."[52] Thus, supporting the cause of socialism was the best the Spanish could do to ensure that "Workers have the right not to suffer tuberculosis, rather than having to be cured by those who have inoculated it."[53]

CONCLUSIONS

Social diseases in Spain, particularly tuberculosis during the Restoration period, are an essential element in understanding the reasons why the so-called social question took the form it did and in coming to terms with its political and ideological impact. The high level of politicization of the health-related aspects of working-class lives came from the clear view that all groups had of the social etiology of diseases. Explicit recognition of poverty as tuberculosis's cause in epidemiological studies of the time was used by socialists as a political weapon, as this cause demonstrated clearly the inequalities between social classes. Hence, the existence of social diseases justified the revolutionary fight and the subversion of the established social order; the solution was to give health and welfare back to the working classes.

In a parallel way, social medicine acquired an essential role in achieving the reformers' aims of ameliorating conditions to counter working-class demands. The goal was to meet the "social problem" with technical solutions that, thanks to their seeming neutrality, would be voluntarily embraced by the working class. Within this process there were also underlying population and regeneration aims – the latter both in its biological and in its moral sense – directed at reaching the state's objective to produce a healthy and an abundant population to nurture the military and the economy.

However, the supporters and practitioners of social medicine experienced difficulties in achieving their socio-political purposes. For example, an emphasis on the depoliticization of tuberculosis, seen in the implementation of bacteriological theories that blamed micro-organisms for the origin of disease and the introduction of sanitary centres, did not find much support within the welfare system. Working-class resistance to medical-social postulates increased because they were supported by the upper middle class, the aristocracy, and the Church, the true *bêtes noires* of the militant working class. From 1913, the organization of the Festival of the Flower was interpreted by many sections of the proletariat as a challenge, showing some of the worst forms of middle-class hypocrisy – collecting from the poor to remedy a problem created in the first place by the actions of the rich. Amongst socialist leaders, "the right to health" was articulated in political terms, being related to all living conditions and not just those targeted by public health officials. The decision by the Partido Socialista Obrero Español (Spanish Working Socialist Party) and the Unión General de Trabajadores (Workers' General Union) to create Red Flower Day to fund *El Socialista* marked the beginning of an organized political response where leaders argued that only the establishment of socialism could produce full health for the whole population. Hence, it is no surprise that early ideas on implementing compulsory health insurance emerged in the anti-tuberculosis congresses. Also, the state eventually decided to undertake social reforms that had been linked to disease prevention from 1917, and the Partido Falangista (Falangist Party) ended up implementing the Seguro Obligatorio de Enfermedad (SOE), or Compulsory Health Insurance, in Spain during the postwar period .[54]

NOTES

The research for this chapter was undertaken within the research project HUM2006–12278–C03–03, funded by the Spanish Ministry of Science and Innovation.

1 Jorge Molero-Mesa, "La tuberculosis como enfermedad social en los estudios epidemiológicos españoles anteriores a la Guerra Civil," *Dynamis* 9 (1989): 185–224.

2 Quoted by Manuel C. Palomeque López, *Derecho del trabajo e ideología: Medio siglo de formación ideológica del Derecho español del trabajo (1873–1923)*, 3d ed. (Madrid: Tecnos 1987), 31–2. See also Antonio Buj Buj, "Inválidos del trabajo: La cuestión sanitaria en los informes de la Comisión de Reformas Sociales," *Scripta Nova, Revista Electrónica de Geografía y Ciencias Sociales*, 6, no. 119 (14) (2002) (http://www.ub.es/geocrit/sn/sn119–14.htm, accessed 5 May 2009).

3 Maria D. de la Calle Velasco, "Sobre los orígenes del Estado social en España," *Ayer* 25 (1997): 127–50. The re-establishment of the Dirección General de Sanidad (National Health Department, 1899), the Law on Women and Children's Work (1900), the Law on Industrial Accidents (1900), the Law on the Protection of Children (1904), the Royal Decree on General Instruction for Public Health (1904), and the creation of the Comisión Permanente de Lucha contra la Tuberculosis (Permanent Commission for the Fight against TB, 1906) were, among others, measures approved during the conservative term of office. See also Santiago Castillo, "Todos iguales ante la ley ... del más fuerte: La legislación laboral y los socialistas españoles en el cambio de siglo (XIX–XX)," *Sociología del Trabajo* 14 (1991–1992): 149–76.

4 Manuel C. Palomeque López, "La intervención normativa del Estado en la cuestión social en la España del siglo XIX," *Ayer* 25 (1997): 103–26.

5 Like some other authors I use variables such as the level of industrialization, the political mobilization of the working class, and constitutional development. However, according to these authors, none of these variables explains the development of social politics that began at the end of the last century in Spain. On the contrary, while they believe it developed out of the "emergence of reformists ideas," such as "liberal krausism, social Catholicism and the confused current of regenerationism," they do not explore the reasons why those ideologies arose. Ana M. Guillén, *El origen del Estado de Bienestar en España (1876–1923): El papel de las ideas en la elaboración de las políticas públicas* (Madrid: Estudios Working Paper, 1990); quoted by Calle Velasco, "Sobre los orígenes," 131.

184 Jorge Molero-Mesa

6 Pedro Carasa Soto, "La pobreza y la asistencia en la historiografía española contemporánea," *Hispania* 50, (1990): 1475–1503; Pedro Carasa Soto, "Metodología del estudio del pauperismo en el contexto de la revolución burguesa española," in S. Castillo (ed.), *La Historia social en España: Actualidad y perspectivas* (Madrid: Siglo XXI, 1991), 359–84; Mariano Esteban de Vega, "Pobreza y beneficencia en la reciente historiografía española," *Ayer* 25 (1997): 15–34; A. Rivera, "Orden social, Reforma social, Estado social," in Santiago Castillo and José Maria Ortiz de Orruño (eds.), *Estado, protesta y movimientos socials* (Bilbao: AHS-U País Vasco 1998), 3–17.

7 Esteban Rodríguez Ocaña, *Por la salud de las naciones: Higiene, Microbiología y Medicina social* (Madrid: Akal 1992). Eugenics was one of the aims of the new social hygiene. About its development in Spain see, Raquel Álvarez, "Eugenesia y control social," *Asclepio* 40 (1988): 29–80; Raquel Álvarez, "Origen y desarrollo de la eugenesia en España," in José Manuel Sánchez Ron (ed.), *Ciencia y sociedad en España: De la Ilustración a la Guerra civil* (Madrid: El Arquero-CSIC 1988), 179–204; Raquel Álvarez, "Penetración y difusión de la eugenesia en España," in Elvira Arquiola and José Martínez (eds.), *Ciencia en expansión: Estudios sobre la difusión de las ideas científicas y médicas en España (siglos XVIII-XX)* (Madrid: Complutense 1995), 211–31. For an overview see Jorge Molero Mesa and Francisco J. Martínez Antonio, "Las campañas sanitarias como paradigma de la acción social de la medicina," *Trabajo Social y Salud* 43 (2002): 119–48.

8 Jorge Molero Mesa, "Francisco Moliner y Nicolás (1851–1915) y el inicio de la Lucha antituberculosa en España," *Asclepio* 42 (1990): 253–80.

9 Esteban Rodríguez Ocaña, "Medicina y acción social en la España del primer tercio del siglo XX," in *De la Beneficencia al Bienestar social: Cuatro siglos de Acción social* (Madrid: Siglo XXI 1986), 227–65; Jorge Molero Mesa, *Estudios medicosociales sobre la tuberculosis en la España de la Restauración* (Madrid: Mº de Sanidad y Consumo 1987); Jorge Molero Mesa, "Fundamentos sociopolíticos de la prevención de la enfermedad en la primera mitad del siglo XX español," *Trabajo Social y Salud* 32 (1999): 19–59; Ricardo Campos Marín, "La sociedad enferma: Higiene y Moral en la segunda mitad del siglo XIX y principios del XX," *Hispania* 55 (1995): 1093–1112; Linda Bryder, *Below the Magic Mountain: A Social History of Tuberculosis in Twentieth-Century Britain* (Oxford: Clarendon Press 1988).

10 Esteban Rodríguez Ocaña and Jorge Molero Mesa, "La cruzada por la salud: Las campañas sanitarias del primer tercio del siglo xx en la construcción de la cultura de la salud," in Luis Montiel (ed.), *La salud en el estado de bienestar: Análisis histórico* (Madrid: Complutense 1993), 133–48.

11 Jorge Molero Mesa, "Los sanatorios para tuberculosos," *El Médico* 501 (1993): 324–34.

12 Alfons Labisch, "Doctors, Workers and the Scientific Cosmology of the Industrial World: The Social Construction of 'Health' and the 'Homo Hygienicus,'" *Journal of Contemporary History* 20 (1985): 599–615; Alfons Labisch, *Homo Hygienicus: Gesundheit und Medizin in der Neuzeit* (Frankfurt: Campus 1992). On the impact of this theory on Spanish historiography see Jorge Molero Mesa, "Del derecho a 'estar sano' al derecho por la 'salud': Socialismo y Medicina social en el primer tercio del siglo xx español," in José Martínez Pérez and Maria I. Porras Gallo (eds.), *Actas del xii Congreso Nacional de Historia de la Medicina, Universidad de Castilla-La Mancha, Albacete 7–9 de febrero de 2002.*

13 Mariano Esteban de Vega, "La asistencia liberal española: Beneficencia pública y previsión particular," *Historia Social* 13 (1992): 123–38.

14 The aim of the present chapter is not an in-depth study of Madrid's tuberculosis epidemiology. For this purpose, see Antonio Fernández García, "La enfermedad como indicador social: Consideraciones metodológicas," in Santiago Castillo (ed.), *La historia social en España: Actualidad y perspectives* (Madrid: Siglo xxi 1990), 401–28; Antonio Fernández García, "Clase obrera y tuberculosis en Madrid a principios del siglo xx," in Rafael Huertas and Ricardo Campos (eds.), *Medicina social y clase obrera en España* (Madrid: FIM 1992), 93–124; Alfredo García Gómez-Álvarez, "La sobremortalidad de la clase obrera madrileña a finales del siglo xix," in Rafael Huertas and Ricardo Campos (eds.), *Medicina social y clase obrera en España* (Madrid: FIM 1992), 145–76; Maria I. Porras Gallo, "Evolución de la mortalidad de Madrid en el periodo 1883–1925: Una aproximación a la realidad sanitaria que conoció Philiph Hauser," in Juan L. Carrillo (ed.), *Entre Sevilla y Madrid: Estudios sobre Hauser y su entorno* (Sevilla: Imp. A. Pinelo 1996), 10–129. On Madrid workers' living conditions between 1898 and 1917 see A. Tiana Ferrer, "La clase obrera en la sociedad madrileña," in *Maestros, misioneros y militantes: La educación de la clase obrera madrileña, 1898–1917* (Madrid: Mº de Educación y Ciencia 1992), 61–112.

15 Vicente Álvarez y Rodríguez-Villamil, *Madrid y la tuberculosis: Memoria presentada al III Congreso Español de la Tuberculosis* (Madrid: Imp. Municipal 1912), 41–2. For the same argument see also Luis Yagüe, "De la alimentación del proletariado en Madrid: Lo que es, lo que debe ser, lo que hoy no puede ser," in *XIV Congres International de medicine, Madrid 23–30 de abril de 1903: Section d'hygiene, epidemiologie et science sanitaire technique* (Madrid: J. Sastre 1904), 96–136, and Esmeralda Ballesteros Doncel, "¡Vivir al límite! Diferencias entre el salario monetario y el presupuesto familiar, siglos XIX y XX," in Santiago Castillo (ed.), *El trabajo a través de la historia : Actas del II Congreso de la Asociación de Historia Social, Córdoba, abril de 1995* (Madrid: Centro de Estudios Históricos UGT-Asociación de Historia Social 1996), 359–66.

16 Juan J. Morato, "El salario y la vida en Madrid," *El Socialista* (8 December 1899).

17 Ricardo Campos Marín, *Alcoholismo, Medicina y Sociedad en España (1876–1923)* (Madrid, CSIC 1997).

18 Quoted by Palomeque López, "La intervención normativa," 123–4.

19 Vicente Guerra y Cortés, *La tuberculosis del proletariado en Madrid* (Madrid: Baena Hermanos 1903), 7.

20 José Codina Castellví, *El problema social de la tuberculosis en Madrid* (Madrid: Enrique Teodoro 1916), 133.

21 "La higiene y las Sociedades Obreras," *El Socialista* (10 November 1899).

22 Between 1900 and 1910, 531 social and labour regulations were enacted in Spain (30 laws, 101 decrees, 356 royal orders, 37 circulars, and 7 different regulations). Palomeque López, "La intervención normativa," 119; see also Demetrio Castro Alfín, "Agitación y orden en la Restauración. ¿Fin del ciclo revolucionario?" *Historia Social* 5 (1989): 37–49.

23 Manuel Pérez Ledesma, "El Estado y la movilización social en el siglo XIX," in Castillo and Ortiz de Orruño, *Estado, protesta*, 215–31.

24 Antonio Espina y Capó, *El Impuesto de consumos y la tuberculosis: Discurso pronunciado en la información oral abierta por la Comisión extraparlamentaria para el estudio de la transformación de este impuesto* (Madrid: Bailly-Baillière e hijos 1906), 8. See full text in Molero Mesa, *Estudios medicosociales*, 107–32.

25 Ibid.

26 Member of the Spanish Parliament and senator throughout his political career, he was director general of public health in 1900.

27 F. Cortajerena y Aldebó, "Acción social moderna ante la tuberculosis," in *III Congreso español de la tuberculosis: Segundo con carácter*

internacional celebrado en San Sebastián 9–16 septiembre 1912, vol. 2
(San Sebastián: Soc. Esp. Papelería 1914), 501–2.

28 De Vega, "La asistencia liberal española."

29 A list of Madrid's charity welfare centres in this period is available in
Marianne Krause, "La beneficencia madrileña en los primeros años del
siglo xx," in *De la Beneficencia*, 267–80.

30 As deduced from workers' testimonies collected by the Social Reforms
Commission in Madrid: Mª.A. Montoya Tamayo and J.C. Frías
Fernández, *La condición obrera hace un siglo: Los trabajadores
madrileños y la Comisión de Reformas Sociales* (Madrid: Universidad
Complutense 1991); see in particular the section "Actitud ante la
beneficencia," 103–7.

31 J. Verdes Montenegro, *La lucha contra la tuberculosis* (Madrid:
Dirección General de Sanidad 1902).

32 Jorge Molero Mesa, "La lucha antituberculosa en España en el primer
tercio del siglo xx," in Juan Atenza and José Martínez Pérez (eds.), *El
Centro Secundario de Higiene Rural de Talavera de la Reina y la Sanidad
Española de su tiempo* (Toledo: Junta de Comunidades de Castilla la
Mancha 2001), 31–147.

33 "Estatutos y Reglamento de la Liga Popular contra la Tuberculosis," in
Trabajos del Real Dispensario Antituberculoso María Cristina de Madrid
(Madrid: Liga Popular contra la Tuberculosis 1912), 404.

34 E. Mesonero Romanos, *La primera fiesta de la Flor (Día de la tuberculosis) celebrada en Madrid, 3 de mayo de 1913: Testimonios que acreditan
que se debió a la iniciativa del doctor Eugenio Mesonero Romanos*
(Madrid: Nicolás Moya 1920).

35 *Gaceta de Madrid* (14 June 1914). The Festival of the Flower was held
until the constitutional government of the Republic abolished it in 1931.
In 1934 Verdes Montenegro, Director General of Public Health during
that year, re-established it. Finally, following the Civil War, it would be
held again from 1945 on.

36 In December of 1918, collector women were officially recognised when
the *Cuerpo de Señoritas Auxiliares de la Doble Cruz Roja* (Body of Assistant Ladies of the Double Red Cross) was created. Among the duties
according to their approved regulations from May 1919 was to help the
Foundation Bodies throughout the year, although the "main mission"
was "collecting on TB Day." "Reglamento del cuerpo de Señoritas
auxiliares de la Doble Cruz Roja," *La Medicina Ibera* 7 (1919), lxxi–ii.

37 "El día de los tuberculosos," *El Socialista,* 18 April 1913.

38 "La fiesta de D. Juan de Robles," *El Socialista,* 4 May 1913.

39 "Crucecitas de flores," *El Socialista,* 1 May 1913.

40 "Cruces, altares y flores," *El Socialista,* 3 May 1913.

41 "El mal del siglo," *El Socialista,* 4 May 1913.

42 "Caridad miserable: Ni a D. Juan de Robles," *El Socialista,* 5 May 1913.

43 "La farsa de las flores," *El Socialista,* 25 November 1913.

44 "Frutos del día de las flores," *El Socialista,* 20 June 1913.

45 "Después de un año: Ni un tuberculoso se ha curado," *El Socialista,* 4 May 1914.

46 "La fiesta de las flores," *El Socialista,* 1 June 1914.

47 E. Fernández, "La fiesta de la Flor Roja," *El Socialista,* 11 April 1915.

48 A. Saborit, "La Fiesta de la Flor Roja," *El Socialista,* 14 April 1915.

49 The first year, it was held in some Asturian localities and in Madrid, where only 150 pesetas were collected. "La actualidad," *El Socialista,* 17 May 1915.

50 "Para Primero de mayo: La flor roja," *El Socialista,* 21 April 1917.

51 "La flor roja," *El Socialista,* 22 April 1915.

52 "Por 'El Socialista': La flor roja," *El Socialista,* 12 June 1916.

53 "Siga la farsa: El escarnio de la miseria," *El Socialista,* 2 June 1915. For an example of Catalan anarchists' rejection of charity medical care, see Isabel Jiménez Lucena and Jorge Molero Mesa, "Per una 'sanitat proletària': L'Organització Sanitària Obrera de la Confederació Nacional del Treball a la Barcelona republicana, (1935–1936)," *Gimbernat* 39 (2003): 211–21.

54 Jorge Molero Mesa and Esteban Rodríguez Ocaña, "Tuberculosis y previsión: Influencia de la enfermedad social modelo en el desarrollo de las ideas médicas españolas sobre el seguro de enfermedad," in *Actas del VIII Congreso Nacional de Historia de la Medicina, Murcia 18–21 diciembre 1986,* vol. 1 (Murcia: Dep. de Historia de la Medicina de la Universidad de Murcia 1988), 502–13; Jorge Molero Mesa, "Health and Public Policy in Spain during the Early Francoist Regime (1936–1951): The Tuberculosis problem," in Illana Löwy and John Krige (eds.), *Images of Disease: Science, Public Policy and Health in Post-war Europe* (Luxembourg: Office for Official Publications of European Commission 2001), 141–65.

9

Lobbying and Resistance with regard to Policy on Bovine Tuberculosis in Britain, 1900–1939: An Inside/Outside Model

PETER J. ATKINS

INTRODUCTION

One of the most interesting and challenging problems related to bovine tuberculosis in Britain in the first half of the twentieth century is explaining the nature of policy-making, its implementation through legislation and regulation, and the outcomes in terms of disease in both animals and humans. Above all, we must account for why it was known and widely accepted in the 1920s and early 1930s that 40 percent of the milking herd was infected, yet why it was not until the 1950s that the radical measures of a major, nationwide slaughter campaign were put in place.

This chapter seeks to understand this slow and tortuous progress of policy by reference to the discursive balance between those activists for and those against change.[1] The struggle between progressive and conservative forces was visible at all levels of the food chain, but the argument here will focus on the voices and actions of selected individuals as representatives of views expressed inside and outside Westminster and Whitehall. My present interest, then, is in agency, although it will become clear that the actions of my case study actors, in both their access to the powerful and their influence upon their decisions, were heavily constrained by the nature and structure of governance.

A widespread distinction is made in the literature on public policy-making between interest groups that have the ear of government and those that are marginalized.[2] First Grant and then

Table 9.1
Categories of Access and Influence

	Inside	Outside
Core	Politicians and others close to decision-making process with strong networks of influence	Reasonably well-connected and resourceful individuals but limited real influence
Peripheral	Politicians and civil servants with intimate knowledge of facts and process but limited power to change policy	Skills, knowledge, with some access and perhaps a media profile but little influence on policy

Maloney, Jordan, and McLaughlin have discussed this distinction as a simple insider/outsider binary, in terms of both status and strategy.[3] Their insights have been valuable but are of limited applicability to this study because they were dealing with Britain after 1945, when the nature and intensity of lobbying by interest groups and the canvassing of opinion by governments had shifted gear. As Martin Smith has pointed out, before 1939 the central state had only loose ties with those wishing to influence policy from outside Westminster, and the present research confirms that policy input from outside was indeed limited for bovine tuberculosis.[4] Where messages did penetrate the consciousness of politicians and civil servants, they tended to be from a relatively small number of sources: a few dairy and medical scientists; farmers' representatives, especially the National Farmers' Union; and a few wealthy individuals who moved in the same social world as the decision makers.

The heterogeneity of access to policy-makers and influence upon them was noticeable, especially in the 1920s and 1930s. For the sake of the present argument, I will reduce this complexity to a stylized distinction between four groups of actors. These groups are derived from a simple 2x2 matrix of inside/outside and core/peripheral (table 9.1).

First, there were what I shall call "core outsiders." These were people with wide interests, abilities, and resources, but limited effectiveness. Like Wilfred Buckley, whose case study I will develop below, they may even have served for a period in government or in an advisory capacity, but the contacts they made were acquaintances rather than friendships or alliances, and their influence was never strong. Buckley, for instance, was used by politicians to trial difficult policies, very much on their terms rather than his. Other examples of core outsiders are Sir William Savage, a medical officer of health and a prolific author on bovine tuberculosis; Sir Graham Selby Wilson, a scientist who championed pasteurization; and Robert Stenhouse Williams, who ran the National Institute for Research in Dairying.[5]

Second, there were "core insiders." Such people may have been high-profile politicians, for example Walter Elliot and Christopher Addison, whose office empowered them to initiate change.[6] Core insiders may also have been lower in profile, like Waldorf Astor, wielding influence directly and indirectly; or they may have been specialists who used narrower channels of access, for example Sir John Boyd Orr, who was originally a laboratory scientist but who became a politician and eventually headed the Food and Agriculture Organization.[7]

Third, we have "peripheral outsiders." There are many possible categories here. Olga Nethersole, the subject of another case study, had no influence but plenty of access. There were some, such as Ben Davies, whose advanced technical expertise was already covered within the circle, and there were others whose views were too extreme or eccentric to allow insider status. Viscount Lymington, who had interests in both agriculture and fascism, was one such.[8]

Fourth, there were the "peripheral insiders," who had less access, less influence, less power. This might have been because of their subordinate role in Whitehall, as was the case with the two civil servants discussed below. It might, as with Sir Edward Grigg, have been because of a tour of duty overseas in the Empire, thus weakening ties at the centre, or it might have been because bovine tuberculosis was only a marginal concern of otherwise senior politicians, such as MPs George Courthope, Sir Edward Strachie, Eleanor Rathbone, and Charles Bathurst.[9]

This chapter will not cover arguments between ministries in Whitehall. They will be discussed elsewhere.[10] Nor will it debate the strategies and tactics of political parties, professional bodies, or lobbying organizations.[11] The concern here is rather with selected individuals who in some way represent a mode of policy-related activity.

In undertaking this approach, I have been influenced by two theoretical literatures beyond policy studies.[12] First, there is what Nigel Thrift has called a non-representational theory that privileges action.[13] His ontological focus is different from mine, yet there is inspiration enough in his notion of "performativity." This notion comes from socio-linguistics in the context of speech acts, the idea there being that performative speech *creates* the truth, but there are also roots in Erving Goffman's interactionist sociology and Judith Butler's identity performances. In the present discussion the concept highlights the activities through which our selected actors attempted, by the deployment of resources, rhetoric, and persuasion to win access to decision makers and influence the policy process.

Second there is the conventions theory of Laurent Thévenot and Luc Boltanski.[14] They are leaders of the French "pragmatic turn" in social theory and their program is an attempt to reconstruct the notion of human action.[15] They are less motivated by an understanding of intentionality than by the constitutive nature of action. For them it is important to build from below a grasp of the way people come to appreciate their commonality and coordinate their efforts into conventions of action. Thévenot and Boltanski are sceptical of any theory of institutional structure that does not take such regimes of engagement into account, and their approach is encouraging for the micro-focus adopted in the present paper because of their interest in the capability and competences that agents bring to any situation of social negotiation.

CORE OUTSIDER: WILFRED BUCKLEY (1873–1933)

The subject of my first case study, Wilfred Buckley, came from a family of wealthy Birmingham merchants.[16] He had no previous farming experience, but in 1906 leased a thousand acres in Hampshire. His interest in clean milk production seems to have been informed by an earlier experience when, in 1902, his daughter had contracted bovine tuberculosis.[17]

Buckley's performance for our purposes was essentially twofold. First, he campaigned for the creation of a clean and honest milk trade, believing that, given the will, it was possible to produce pure milk, without added water and without the germs of infectious disease. Although this idea is taken for granted amongst the public in Britain today, to many at the beginning of the twentieth century it seemed idealistic to the point of naivety. Because the structural and procedural changes that Buckley advocated for the cowshed would have been expensive to implement, he became the *bête noir* of farmers and the milk trade, who branded him a dilettante. One trade paper went further: "in a word Mr Buckley is the enemy."[18]

It is not difficult to see why farmers resented Buckley's views. In 1924, for instance, he wrote to the Ministry of Agriculture (MAF) arguing that no compensation should be given to farmers for the compulsory slaughter of diseased cattle under the Tuberculosis Order because "a producer is acting immorally in selling milk from a cow that is suffering from the diseases enumerated in the Order."[19] He argued instead for cattle insurance. In his moral crusade, one might have thought that Buckley was most likely to find common cause with consumers, but one of his unlikely allies was Ben Davies, a director of one the largest dairy corporations, United Dairies. Talking about clean and disease-free production methods, Davies argued that it was farmers who should bear the responsibility. "Those surely are merely the fundamental decencies of the production of human food, and failure to observe them must be regarded as a culpable and penal offence involving even disqualification as a producer."[20]

Second, in essence, Buckley's public life was devoted to the translation of American methods of clean milk production into the British sphere. He had married an American heiress and made regular business visits to New York connected with his family's trading company. He was therefore in a privileged position to see innovations in action and to judge their suitability for the somewhat different conditions on this side of the Atlantic.

His principal platform was as the co-founder and Chairman of the National Clean Milk Society (NCMS), (1915–28). The aim of this organization was educational: producing pamphlets, distributing films and lantern slides, mounting exhibits at agricultural shows, and holding lectures, mainly given by Buckley himself in every part of the country. He opposed legislation as coercive, claiming to prefer persuasion.[21] The council of the NCMS was comprised of the great and the good, including the King's surgeon, Sir Frederick Treves, and a number of other doctors.

Buckley's farm became a showcase for his ideas. In 1910–11 a committee chaired by Sir Thomas Barlow, president of the Royal College of Physicians, undertook practical experiments there on clean milk production. Their recommendation to the Local Government Board was the adoption of the American-style system of milk certification for cleanliness advocated by Buckley. The inclusion of an enabling provision in the Milk and Dairies Act of 1914 was a direct outcome.[22] A related American idea was the "score card

system" of judging the cleanliness of milk production, first introduced in the District of Columbia in 1904.[23] Buckley's enthusiasm
for the system eventually persuaded the city authorities in Birmingham and Bradford to try it in 1915 and from there it spread.

Buckley is interesting and unusual because of his total focus on
the issue. He seems to have been unconcerned about party or class-
based politics and was oblivious to criticism. Just before he died of
cancer in 1933, he reminisced that 1912–13 had been a turning
point in his activist career. He had been unable to get support from
his richer friends, "but when I went to the Labour people I got help.
Henderson said: 'the crumbs will drop from the rich man's table.'
That is the expression he used, and that is why the Labour Party
adopted the idea of grades of milk."[24] These contacts bore fruit
when in August 1917 he was asked by Lord Rhondda to become
director of milk supplies at the Ministry of Food. Very quickly he
managed to persuade his patron to allow licences and higher prices
for hygienic producers. Lord Rhondda died before the regulations
came into force, but the new food controller, John Clynes, was
favourable, and grading was established.

Wilfred Buckley had enemies not only in the dairy industry but
also in Whitehall. The chief veterinary officer, Stuart Stockman,
was particularly scathing about his opposition to compensation for
the slaughter of tuberculous cattle: "He has got his own Grade A
herd, achieved without compensation, earning premium for milk,
so doesn't want too many competitors."[25] Such cynicism was almost
certainly misplaced, but Buckley does not seem to have been sensi-
tive to the public perception of his actions.

For all of his commitment and energy, Buckley was certainly not
a sophisticated political operator. As chairman of a sub-committee
of the Astor Committee in 1918 he recommended the nationalisa-
tion of the wholesale milk trade.[26] This recommendation appealed
to the food controller but to virtually no-one else, and it lasted only
six months.[27] The following year he was involved in a major spat
over milk prices. His committee had imposed a zonal pricing system
in which farmers would be paid less in the South West zone, where
costs of production were said to be lower. Any milk travelling from
one zone to another was to pass through a government-controlled
clearing house. But this system was over-complicated, and anyway
information about the costs of production was scarce because most
farmers did not keep records. There was even talk of consumers

having to register and of milk delivery rounds being rationalized. This time Buckley was forced to resign; although as a face-saving measure he stayed on as a technical adviser on milk to the Ministry of Food until it was finally wound up in March 1921.[28]

Buckley may have been unsuccessful as a civil servant but he was in his element as a committee man. He seems to have been involved on a voluntary basis in most of the milk-related committees that mattered in the decade or so after the First World War. I have already mentioned his role in the Astor Committee, and to this we might add the Tuberculin Committee (jointly sponsored by the Medical Research Council (MRC) and the Agricultural Research Council), by which his farm was used to judge whether the tuberculin test would affect the fat content of milk.[29] In addition, he was a member of the Inter-Departmental Committee on Condensed Milk, 1920. He was a founding member of the National Milk Publicity Council (NMPC) in the same year, its chairman from 1922 to 1924, and a leading light in its encouragement of school milk in 1928. From 1924 he was a member of the government's Milk Advisory Committee (MAC). He also somehow found the time to organize a series of high-profile annual National Milk Conferences, 1922–24, which discussed clean milk, tuberculosis, and pasteurization, and, out of government, he made visits to ministers as a member of several official delegations on the subject of milk.[30]

Buckley was also a frequent letter writer. Much of his output was directed to prominent individuals or to the Ministries of Agriculture and Health; the *Times* and the *Observer* were other favoured outlets, especially for his views on the need for both the milk trade and their customers to be educated on the requirement for a better standard of product.[31] The opinions expressed were at times radical, for instance in 1912 when he wrote to the *Times* arguing that pasteurization was not necessary if milk was produced in clean conditions from tuberculin-tested cattle. This was vintage Buckley, in a sense stating the obvious but ignoring the practical difficulties in achieving the ideal.

Overall, Buckley was very active across a wide range of performances (table 2). He was used by Lloyd George's government as a lightning conductor for difficult policies, and he never shirked controversy.[32] Buckley used his contacts in political circles to move his agenda forward, but he lacked several of the resources cited by Keith Dowding as a *sine qua non* for powerful bargaining:

Table 9.2
A Summary of Performances

	Buckley	Astor	Nethersole	Dale & Blackshaw
Personal contacts	✓	✓	✓	✓
Media	✓		✓	
Official debates		✓	✓	
Delegations to ministries	✓		✓	
Parliamentary committees	✓	✓		✓
Whitehall bureaucracy	✓	✓		✓
Quangos	✓			
Trade and professional	✓			
Private societies	✓	✓	✓	

legitimate authority, incentives to affect the interests of others, and an unchallenged reputation.[33]

CORE INSIDER: WALDORF ASTOR (1879–1952)

Waldorf Astor was not a high-profile politician. According to a perceptive comment in the *Dictionary of National Biography*, "he was a committee man, rather than an individualist, and for this reason his influence on affairs was not always easy to trace." He is probably best known for being the son of a wealthy New York property developer, husband of Britain's first female member of Parliament, and host of the Nazi appeasers, the Cliveden set.[34] I want to argue that we should attribute to him achievements in his own right in the area of milk and tuberculosis policy.

Astor was unable to serve in the First World War because of the bovine tuberculosis that he is said to have caught in 1905. Nevertheless, he busied himself as Unionist MP for Plymouth (1911–19), then in the House of Lords as Viscount Astor when his father died. He was a member of the Round Table Group of Conservative MPs, along with Ned Grigg, later one of the architects of a new milk marketing system, and he was appointed parliamentary secretary to Lloyd George in 1917, parliamentary secretary to the Ministry of Food in 1918, parliamentary secretary in the Ministry of Health from 1919 to 1921, and, later, British delegate to League of Nations in 1931.[35] As proprietor of the *Observer*, Astor was in a position to exert considerable influence. He frequently published letters and articles on tuberculosis by the likes of Wilfred Buckley, despite the occasional protests of his editor.[36]

Although on some policy issues a social radical, nevertheless Astor was by political instinct a gradualist. A quotation from his writings in 1920 illustrates this point: "It would be almost criminal folly to try to improve the whole [milk] supply quickly by coercion. We should drive too many farmers out of business. What we want to do is to set out to encourage improvement ... over a period of, say, 10 to 15 years."[37] His program for the reduction of bovine tuberculosis was very similar to Buckley's. They both advocated graded milk, to which Astor added ideas about "attested herds" and free milk for women entitled to maternity benefit.[38]

Waldorf Astor made an important contribution as a chairman of parliamentary committees. In 1912 he chaired the Local Government Board's important Departmental Committee on Tuberculosis.[39] This was set up to make practical suggestions arising from the scientific work of the Royal Commission that finished its work and reported in 1911. One of their principal recommendations was the establishment of a Medical Research Committee, whose task would be to organize and promote research on tuberculosis.[40] One can see Astor's hand in the declaration by his committee that "the ultimate eradication of animal tuberculosis is not impossible of achievement, but is likely to be a slow process."

The second Astor Committee, sitting from 1917 to 1919, was another departmental committee, this time on the Production and Distribution of Milk.[41] Here he highlighted a possible accredited herd scheme based on recent American experience.[42] There were also recommendations to improve tuberculin testing: the manufacture of the tuberculin by the government laboratory at Weybridge; the standardization of the tuberculin dose; and free testing for farmers entering an accreditation scheme. A version of the accredited herd idea was eventually implemented in the form of "Attested Herds" from 1935 onwards, when it became the most important single policy move towards the elimination of bovine tuberculosis. But in 1919 it was not practical politics, and, anyway, the committee's positive achievements were soon overshadowed by the political crisis of milk prices in the winter of 1918–19, mentioned above, and by an avalanche of criticism of its advocacy of state participation in both the wholesale and the retail milk trades.

In 1920 Waldorf Astor, who by then was parliamentary secretary at the Ministry of Health, arranged for a £1,000 one-off grant to the National Clean Milk Society, of which both he and Buckley were patrons. This rather naïf piece of favouritism cannot have endeared him to many, and it is perhaps not surprising that in 1922 and 1923, when Whitehall was looking for a chairman for its new MAC, he was passed over in favour of "someone who was more independent."[43] This was the time (1922–24) when he was president of the NMPC and therefore could be said to have had an axe to grind.[44]

Out of government Astor was an energetic and astute lobbyist. He seems to have concentrated on four groups of contacts. First, there were medical scientists who had knowledge of tuberculosis and could therefore add weight to his own lay views. An example is Dr C.J. Martin, the director of the Lister Institute of Preventive Medicine, whom in 1914 Astor asked to write letters to the *Times* and an article in the *New Statesman*. Then there were several influential rural MPs and members of the House of Lords who were interested in milk and disease and who were approached for their opinions or persuaded to vote on a particular bill. Astor was also regularly in touch with senior civil servants, such as Sir Arthur Robinson of the Ministry of Health, who in 1923 asked him to act as an intermediary with the Labour Party leaders over the Milk and Dairy (Amendment) Bill, which they were opposing because it did not go far enough over certified milk. Finally, there were occasional private meetings with ministers throughout the 1920s and 1930s.[45]

Deploying his contacts in the latter two categories, Astor's lobbying certainly forced a response in Whitehall. In 1925 he was particularly exercised by milk grading, the only means by which the public could distinguish disease-free milk. In July he told Sir George Newman, chief medical officer of the Ministry of Health, that he was unhappy with the grades then in operation and that he was planning a deputation to the minister or questions in the House of Lords.[46] While politicians and civil servants seem to have favoured a simplification of the grades at that point, they were conscious that milk had been such a difficult political issue over the previous fifteen years or so and had a clear preference for a quiet Whitehall compromise rather than an open debate: "The only way to get a satisfactory solution to a question of this kind is to confer with the parties interested. A formal deputation to the Minister is not the way to get down to the problem – still less questions in parliament

... I think if you could tell Lord Astor that an informal conference with him and his friends would be the best way of opening the ball it would be advisable to do so."[47]

Astor was quietly invited to the Ministry and brought with him Wilfred Buckley and George Dallas, a Labour MP who specialised in food and agriculture issues. Their opening salvo was that "the Ministry had been negligent in the milk question."[48] After that they proposed a new set of grades and demanded that local authorities should be allowed to make labelling, bottling, and pasteurization compulsory in their own districts if they so wished.[49] This was effectively the program of the NCMS, of which Astor and Buckley were the leading lights. Lest he should be mistaken for a dewy-eyed romantic, Astor later wrote to Neville Chamberlain, then minister of health, stressing that he thought his staged plan was realistic: "Ideally all milk sold should be officially labelled. Everyone would then know what he was buying. It is not practical politics to do this now for the whole country, but the aim of the government should be to reach such a policy in say 10–15 years time."[50]

The Ministries of Health and Agriculture held a meeting at the level of parliamentary secretary (Lord Bledisloe for Agriculture and Sir H. Kingsley Wood for Health) to discuss Astor's intervention. They concluded that for numerous reasons his scheme was unworkable. One reason was the logistical problem of organizing a nationwide system of bacteriological sampling. Another was that "the time is not yet ripe for any alteration with regard to Grade 'A' milk." They preferred instead to put their faith in a propaganda drive to "create a public opinion in favour of clean milk, and a public demand for it."[51]

In sum, what was Astor's achievement? I suggest that he did as much as any politician in the period 1900–39 (other than Christopher Addison and Walter Elliot) to get milk onto the health agenda. He did not seek out the newspaper headline writers but made countless discreet interventions in Whitehall, Westminster, and beyond and acted as a catalyst for change.

PERIPHERAL OUTSIDER: OLGA NETHERSOLE (1870–1951)

Olga Nethersole was an actress-manager who made a good living at the turn of the century from what at the time were considered somewhat risqué plays. Upon retirement she was involved with the Red

Cross in the First World War and in 1917 founded the People's League of Health (PLH) with the aim of encouraging preventative medicine. She started campaigning proper in 1920, and her first interest in bovine tuberculosis seems to have been in 1929.[52] Margaret Barnett has written at length on Nethersole's efforts in this direction, concluding that on balance they were positive.[53] I want to add further thoughts on her influence and impact.

Nethersole must have been a very persuasive person because she attracted dozens of participants to PLH committees and as general supporters. The famous "Survey of Tuberculosis of Bovine Origin," formally published in January 1932, for instance, is prefaced with lists of supporters. In addition to the patronage of King George V, there were nineteen titled vice-presidents, a medical council of ninety-one, and a general bovine tuberculosis committee of sixty-five, including Wilfred Buckley.[54] Given Nethersole's recruitment methods, some of these people were not very active, and a few were apparently even surprised to see their names mentioned. Arguably, most names were little more than bunting, just there for show. Nevertheless, the three sub-committees that actually prepared the raw material for the survey and then wrote the report were made up of those who were truly at the forefront of knowledge and activism on bovine tuberculosis: medical men (William Savage, William Hunter), scientists (Graham Selby Wilson, James Macintosh, Jack Drummond, Norman Wright, and Robert Stenhouse Williams), politicians (Sir Archibald Weighall), and milk traders (Edward Freeth and James Sadler). This was a resource of big-hitters the like of which had rarely been assembled as witnesses to an official enquiry such as a royal commission, let alone a private and purely voluntary effort organized by one woman.

Olga Nethersole may have been exceptionally good at networking, but she faced opposition. One example will suffice. In March 1930, Stanley Griffiths, one of the most prominent laboratory researchers on tuberculosis, wrote to his employer, Walter Fletcher, secretary of the MRC. Griffiths had received an invitation from the PLH to serve on its bovine tuberculosis committee. He was afraid that it would interfere with his work and sought advice.[55] The reply is revealing: "I am afraid I know all about this People's League, and it is becoming a great nuisance. It is sheer impertinence to ask you to waste your time in the manner proposed, with a mixed lot of charlatans and advertisers (with one or two honest men who have been had for mugs and ought to have known better). I not only think you're right in refusing, but I think you ought to refuse."[56]

Later he urged Griffiths to "tell Olga Nethersole to go to blazes."[57] Fletcher also wrote to a number of his associates to warn them that the MRC did not approve of the PLH.

> I note your name as a member of a fantastic "sub-committee on bovine tuberculosis" appointed by the People's League of Health. This thing was due to an agitation by a tiresome busy-body called [Dr Gordon] Tippett, reacting upon dear Miss Nethersole, who *is* the League of Health. It is an absurdity because it is composed of 30 to 40 persons, most of whom know nothing of the subject at first hand. It has grown just as snowballs do grow, man after man being flattered by Miss Nethersole into joining, and each name being used to catch others. I am disturbed by seeing your name as a member. This embarrasses us.[58]

A similar attitude was taken at the Ministry of Health, where the permanent secretary instructed that "Miss O. Nethersole should be put in her place, with firmness but with the politeness customary to you."[59]

It is worth recalling that this was a very active period in the history of policy-making on bovine tuberculosis. There was an interdepartmental committee in 1930/31.[60] In 1931 there was a short debate in the House of Lords, memorable mainly for a powerful speech on the need for change by Lord Moynihan of Leeds, president of Royal College of Surgeons.[61] The MRC launched three relevant reports between 1930 and 1933.[62] In 1932 the Reorganization Commission on Milk began its deliberations and took evidence on disease and heat treatment, and the Gowland Hopkins Committee met for the first time, leading up to the publication of its report in 1934.[63] In 1933 the City of Manchester held a referendum on the subject of pasteurization, showing the extraordinary depth of feeling on this potential method of protecting the public.[64] In short, there was a ferment of ideas about policy options, and the PLH report represented an opportunity for those already engaged in this debate to fire another salvo, to the discomfort of the vested interests at the MRC and the Ministry of Health. Nethersole provided a convenient platform at just the right time. There was little that was new in the report of the PLH, but it undoubtedly made an impact, judging from the frequent citations in the media and various political fora.

The PLH continued until 1950, although it had long since lost its voice and had fallen into debt.[65] Apart from this one brief triumph and one or two other notorious excursions into health politics, it was largely ineffective in political terms, apart from being a general irritant in Whitehall. The PLH is an example of what we might call a "pseudo network," one without real depth, without rhizomic power.

PERIPHERAL INSIDERS: J.F. BLACKSHAW AND H.E. DALE

All the actors discussed so far were busy and effective to one degree or another. However, their impact was limited: graded milk was very slow to be adopted, compulsory pasteurization was delayed, and, as milk consumption expanded in the 1930s, the risk of tuberculosis increased. Was it that progressives were swimming in a sea of indifference, or was it that they were meeting organized resistance? No and yes.

As I have shown in other papers, the opposition to the changes (legislative, technical) that would have reduced the risk of bovine tuberculosis was comprised of ideologues and vested interests.[66] The former were mainly in the anti-pasteurization camp (organicists, etc.), the latter in the farming industry and parts of the milk trade. Throughout the early twentieth century, food and milk were never political priorities, and it was therefore relatively easy to disrupt any legislation that came forward. Labour was the only political party to take milk seriously, but their periods in office were short, and even during the first National Government (1931–35) Ramsay MacDonald gave the Ministries of Agriculture and Health to Conservatives.

A major shift came in 1933 when Walter Elliot set up the Milk Marketing Board as a corporate institution dominated by the farmers. He ceded power to them, making reforms by the Ministry of Agriculture & Fisheries (MAF) even more difficult. It took reforms in the Second World War, the Labour victory in 1945, and Tom Williams, a dedicated minister of agriculture, to start genuine and fundamental change.

What was the performance of the MAF in the 1920s and 1930s? It is best summed up in the activities of two figures in nodal bureaucratic positions: J.F. Blackshaw, dairy commissioner, and H.E. Dale, principal assistant secretary. A very crude encapsulation of their views on radical change to eliminate bovine tuberculosis would have been: it can't be done because it is too big a problem, change would damage the farming industry, and the science is uncertain. In these arguments they were entraining and translating the "interests" of farmers and farm animals and drawing very considerable strength from the lobbying of agricultural groups. They showed no grasp of what today we call the precautionary principle, the principle that, where unambiguous proof of cause and effect is not available, it is necessary to act with a duty of care.

Although they were on every relevant committee in Whitehall and many outside, Blackshaw and Dale are mainly visible in the private papers of the MAF in the National Archives. The hand-written "minutes" are often the most revealing. Here are three quotations that make this point.

Dale (1932): If one admits the evil [of bovine tuberculosis], the question is, is the means suggested for dealing immediately with it likely to produce more or less evil in the long run to the community? If you get 5,000 or 10,000 or 15,000 people [farmers] ruined, what is going to be the effect on the wives and children of those men?[67]

Blackshaw (1933): So far as I can see, if tuberculosis were eradicated universally by all farmers equally it is at least doubtful whether there would be any gain to the industry. The cost of producing milk would presumably be reduced, but if the reduction were universal it would merely mean that pretty soon the price would fall and everyone except the customer would be where he was before.[68]

Blackshaw (1934): It is perhaps a pity that these people [the PLH], as well as the [Hopkins] committee, persisted in looking at this matter from the platform of the idealist and not the platform of the practical possibilist. In my view it would not be practicable at the present time to require that all milk produced for consumption must be of Grade A standard when it leaves the farm. Any attempt to administer such a regulation in the present state of affairs would quickly result in a milk shortage.[69]

In short, these civil servants used every opportunity open to them, both in outside committees and behind closed doors in the ministry, to prevent costly change. The Ministry of Health dubbed Blackshaw and Dale "the more old fashioned part of the Ministry [of Agriculture]," and there seems to have been a collective sigh of relief when they both retired in 1935.[70] Their careers were a testament to the effectiveness of what Michel de Certeau would have recognised as their everyday tactical resistance.[71]

DISCUSSION

Bob Jessop sees the state as a "site, generator and product of strategies." In his view "any theory of the state must produce an informed analysis of the strategic calculations and practices of the actors involved and of the interaction between agents and the state structures. However the relationship is always dynamic and dialectical."[72] The present chapter has attempted to add a further layer of understanding to recent reconstructions of the complex nature of bovine tuberculosis policy-making in Britain before the Second World War. There is a risk, however, that such a short chapter might give the impression of a reductive view of state action. It is therefore important to make two cautionary points.

First, the slow advance in policy with regard to bovine tuberculosis did not mean a lack of progress across the board. Several initiatives *were* undertaken by government, although most improvements came from the commercial world. Graded milk, for instance, was introduced in 1917 and relaunched in 1923, although it did not have much impact in our period.[73] There was also the idea of attested herds, which was altogether more significant, starting a year or two before the Second World War. Finally, and most important, pasteurization was introduced gradually by dairy companies in the inter-war period. This method of heat treatment was primarily designed to increase the shelf life of retail milk, but in its technically most efficient guises, it had the beneficial side effect of killing the mycobacteria that had been passed on by infectious cows.

Second, the local state was heavily involved in making and implementing policy with regard to bovine tuberculosis. My discussion here has been London-focused, but a fully nuanced model must account for the geographically uneven responses of local authorities, with large cities such as Manchester, Liverpool, and Glasgow in the lead.[74]

I see the next step in this research as accommodating the view of Marsh and Smith that policy studies must move beyond the structure/agency dichotomy.[75] Actor network theory, or what in Deleuzian terms has been renamed actant rhizomic theory, provides a convenient and well-tried means of taking interest networks seriously as agents in their own right. ANT sets aside binary oppositions such as inside/outside and deals instead with heterogeneous associations: networks made up of people, technology, animals. For Bruno Latour's laboratory scientists, their ability to put their ideas forward and exert influence depends upon their resources of hardware, their working methods, their network of contacts. My campaigners for action with regard to bovine tuberculosis needed to entrain wide networks of different actors in order to get their way. Actors build networks by translating the interests of others into their own cause. This may involve hybrids of social and natural phenomena, for instance representing the interests of cattle in a debate about a zoonosis. Campaigners can therefore be seen as speaking on behalf of both people and animals.

In the context of a different cattle disease, bovine spongiform encephalopathy (BSE), Steve Hinchliffe has looked at what is involved in making a policy decision. His conclusion involves the extent to which nature can be known and the knowing of indeterminacy. Significantly, the science of BSE/CJD has proved to be slippery and uncertain in a way that is very reminiscent of bovine tuberculosis. The time scales and many of the details of the two zoonoses are rather different, yet Hinchliffe's commentary on policy-making is highly relevant also for bovine tuberculosis: "The production of a policy is a struggle to align all manner of people, utterances, departments and knowledges ... A ... policy does not ... survive or fall on its own merits. It is a networked achievement."[76]

CONCLUSION

The accompanying figure (9.1) sketches the actor space of policy-making with regard to bovine tuberculosis. It shows some of the interrelationships that I have discussed, but it is not a power map. Complex versions of such relationship diagrams have been subjected to

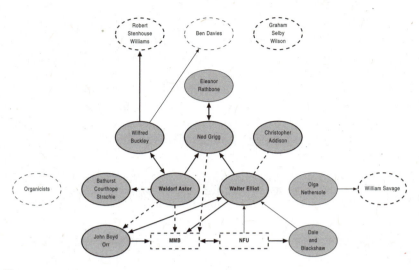

Figure 9.1
The actor space of policy-making

mathematical network analysis by sociologists, and it is interesting
to note that a software industry has recently emerged to assist corporations concerned about the efficiency of interaction amongst
their staff.[77]

My conclusion is that bovine tuberculosis lived and thrived in a
relational world. Delays in policy formation were caused by the
inability of actors such as Buckley, Astor, and Nethersole to make
the necessary extensions of their projects into the parts of Whitehall
that mattered. In addition, there was no meeting of minds. Dale and
Blackshaw had no empathy with consumer causes, because they felt
that they themselves were employed solely to protect the farming
industry. What they apparently could not see was that the interests
of farming were to an extent bound up with creating trust in the
food chain. This issue is still crucial today.

The balance between progressives and conservatives remained
very much in the favour of the latter camp throughout our period.
However, the Second World War broke the log-jam, with the capacity of conservative politicians and civil servants greatly reduced,
and the situation after 1945 was different again. There was much
closer collaboration between the governments and interest groups,
and the political will to slaughter large numbers of infected cattle
around the country reached its peak in the 1950s.

My insider/outsider classification of activism has served its purpose, but further work will stress the interweaving of individual and group projects. It remains to be seen whether there is clearer evidence of networked achievements in policy-making than has been shown in the present chapter.

NOTES

1 I am grateful to the Wellcome Trust for the financial support provided for the research for this chapter and to the other delegates at the Sheffield Conference for their constructive criticism my paper.

2 David Marsh and Rob A.W. Rhodes (eds.), *Policy Networks in British Governance* (Oxford: Clarendon Press 1992); Rob A.W. Rhodes, *Understanding Governance: Policy Networks, Governance, Reflexivity and Accountability* (Buckingham: Open University Press 1997); Wyn Grant, *Pressure Groups and British Politics* (Basingstoke: Macmillan 2000); Mark Bevir and Rod A.W. Rhodes, *Interpreting British Governance* (London: Routledge 2003).

3 Wyn Grant, "Insider Groups, Outsider Groups and Interest Group Strategies in Britain," *University of Warwick Department of Politics Working Paper* No. 19 (1978); William A. Maloney, Grant Jordan, and Andrew M. McLaughlin, "Interest Groups and Public Policy: the Insider/Outsider Model Revisited," *Journal of Public Policy* 14 (1994):17–38.

4 Martin J. Smith, *The Politics of Agricultural Support in Britain: The Development of the Agricultural Policy Community* (Aldershot: Dartmouth 1990).

5 William Savage (1872–1961) was medical officer of health for Somerset, Graham Wilson (1895–1987) developed laboratory methods of testing milk quality, and Robert Williams (1871–1932) was a prominent advocate of clean milk production.

6 Walter Elliot (1888–1959) and Christopher Addison (1869–1951), later Viscount Addison, during their careers were both ministers of health and ministers of agriculture.

7 John Orr (1880–1971), later Lord Boyd-Orr, was an MP for the brief period of 1945–46.

8 Viscount Lymington (1898–1984) later became the Earl of Portsmouth.

9 Grigg (1879–1955), later Baron Altrincham, was governor of Kenya 1925–30; George Courthope (1877–1955), later Baron Courthope; Sir Edward Strachie (1858–1936); Eleanor Rathbone (1872–1946); and Charles Bathurst (1867–1958), later Viscount Bledisloe.

10 Peter J. Atkins, "White Heat in Whitehall: Inter-departmental Friction and Its Impact upon Food Safety Policy, the Example of Milk, 1930–35," unpublished ms., 2006c.

11 Peter J. Atkins, "'Your Enemy the Cow': Actors, Networks and Competitive Interests in the Medical, Veterinary and Administrative Debate about Bovine Tuberculosis in Britain, circa 1800–1964," unpublished ms., 2006a.

12 These two theoretical contexts informed my preliminary thinking about the scale at which to pitch my analysis and the emphasis upon activities rather than structures. I do not, in this paper at least, adopt their vocabulary or their epistemologies.

13 Nigel Thrift, "Steps to an Ecology of Place," in Doreen Massey, John Allen, and Phil Sarre (eds.), *Human Geography Today* (Cambridge: Polity Press 1999), 295–322.

14 Luc Boltanski and Laurent Thévenot, *De la Justification* (Paris: Gallimard 1991); Laurent Thévenot, "Pragmatic Regimes Governing the Engagement with the World," in Theodore R. Schatzki, Karin Knorr Cetina, and and Eike von Savigny (eds.), *The Practice Turn in Contemporary Theory* (London: Routledge 2001), 56–73.

15 Thomas Bénatouïl, "A Tale of Two Sociologies: The Critical and the Pragmatic Stance in Contemporary French Sociology," *European Journal of Social Theory* 2 (1999): 379–96; Peter Wagner, *A History and Theory of the Social Sciences* (London: Sage 2001).

16 Obituaries: *The Times*, 28 October 1933, 7, and 1 November 7; *Milk Industry* 14 (1933), 84.

17 Philip Sheail, "Hampshire Man and the Quest for Clean Milk," *Hampshire* (March 1981): 60–2.

18 *The Dairyman, the Cowkeeper, and Dairyman's Journal* (January 1919):101.

19 National Archives (NA): MAF 35/309. Tuberculosis Orders were used as a means of the compulsory slaughter of diseased animals.

20 B. Davies, "Practical and Scientific Problems of the Milk Supply and Their Laboratory Control," *Journal of the Royal Sanitary Institute* 54 (1934):486–501, 488.

21 Wilfred Buckley, "Limits of Pasteurization: Better Milk Means More Business," *The Milk Industry* 2, 8 (February 1922):79–81.

22 This gave powers to the Local Government Board to designate and regulate certified milk. The postponement of this legislation in 1915 was a disappointment.

23 The cleanliness of the following items was scored: cows, cowshed, utensils, the milk room, and milking and milk handling methods.

24 NA: CAB 58/186, Economic Advisory Council, Report, Proceedings and Memoranda of Committee on Cattle Diseases (EAC (CD) Series, 88–109A), 1932–34, vol. 3, Memorandum no. 99: Stenographic notes of the evidence of Wilfred Buckley.

25 NA: MAF 35/309.

26 Departmental Committee on the Production and Distribution of Milk, 1917–19.

27 Wholesale Milk Dealers (Control) Order 1918, *Statutory Rules and Orders* no. 24.

28 There were further controversial episodes in the 1920s: for instance in 1926 Buckley gave evidence to the Food Council that short measure was endemic. This caused such an outcry in the milk trade that the farmers and retailers demanded that he should repudiated by the NMPC for whom he was then working. When the latter refused, the relationship between the National Farmers Union and the NMPC deteriorated to breaking point. NA: MAF/52/7, TD/428.

29 NA: MH 56/110.

30 For instance, twice in March 1914 he made visits to the Local Government Board as a delegate of the Agricultural Organization Society and then the Barlow Committee arguing for milk certification. NA: MH 80/5.

31 Waldorf Astor was proprietor of the *Observer* and was therefore predisposed to giving Buckley a voice because of his own interest in milk.

32 One example of his boldness was his appointment as organizer-in-chief of London's milk supply during the General Strike of 1926.

33 Keith Dowding, "Model or Metaphor? A Critical Review of the Policy Network Approach," *Political Studies* 43 (1995):136–58.

34 His father was William Waldorf Astor, owner of the Waldorf Astoria hotel, and his wife was Nancy Astor.

35 In 1936 he became chairman of the Joint Committee of Agricultural, Economic and Health Experts appointed by the League, which later became the Food and Agriculture Organization of the United Nations.

36 University of Reading Archives, Astor Papers, MS1066/1/1023.

37 Waldorf Astor, "The Production of Pure Milk," *The Farmers' Union Year Book*, section 7 (1920/21): 1–6.

38 Reading University Archives, Astor Papers: MS1066/1/1019; *Parliamentary Debates* 61 (1914) 1023–67.

39 Waldorf Astor (chairman), Departmental Committee on Tuberculosis, Interim Report, British Parliamentary Papers 1912–13 (Cd 6164), xlviii.1; Final Report, British Parliamentary Papers 1912–13 (Cd 6641), xlviii. 29; Appendix, British Parliamentary Papers 1912–13 (Cd 6654), xlviii.47.

40 Christopher Addison was a member of the Departmental Committee, and both he and Astor were on the subsequent Medical Research Committee.

41 Waldorf Astor (chairman), Departmental Committee on Production and Distribution of Milk, *First Interim Report,* British Parliamentary Papers 1917–18 (Cd 8608), xvi.1003; *Second Interim Report*, British Parliamentary Papers 1917–18 (Cd 8886), xvi.1011; *Third Interim Report,* British Parliamentary Papers 1919 (Cmd 315), xxv.615; *Final Report*, British Parliamentary Papers 1919 (Cmd 483), vvx.645.

42 This would have meant payments to farmers for milk of a higher than average bacteriological quality.

43 NA: MH 56/75, 23 October 1923, Floud to Robinson.

44 His only other official work in this area came in 1934 when he chaired a Milk Marketing Board committee advising on activities involving expenditure under the Milk Act (1934) for milk publicity and school milk.

45 The best source for these various activities is the Astor Papers in the University of Reading Archives.

46 Astor wanted a hierarchy of grades, such as A, B, and C, rather than grades of vague relative merit, such as Grade A and Certified.

47 NA: MH/56/77. R.B. Cross, undated minute [July 1925].

48 NA: MH/56/77. Memo from Newman, 16 July 1925. 'Negligent' here referred to the continuing loss of life from tuberculosis and the need for a tightening of the regulations.

49 NA: MH/56/77. Letter from Lord Astor to Sir George Newman, 11 July 1925. There were to be six grades in the proposed system, ranked according to bacteriological quality and whether the milk had been tuberculin tested and pasteurized. Coloured milk tops were to be used as markers for the consumer.

50 NA: MH/56/77. Astor to Chamberlain, 31 July 1925, with the salutation "Dear Neville."

51 NA: MH/56/77. Memo by Beckett, 16 September 1925, Beckett summarising the meeting between Lord Bledisloe and Sir Kingsley Wood.

52 NA: FD 1/1649.

53 Margaret Barnett, "The People's League of Health and the Campaign against Bovine Tuberculosis in the 1930s," in David F. Smith and Jim Phillips (eds.), *Food, Science, Policy and Regulation in the Twentieth Century: International and Comparative Perspectives* (London: Routledge 2000), 69–82.

54 The Medical Council comprised a formidable list of surgeons, physicians, and medical officers of health, including one lord, one lady, twenty-five knights and six professors.

55 NA: FD 1/1649. Griffiths to Fletcher, 13 March 1930.

56 NA: FD 1/1649. Fletcher to Griffiths, 17 March 1930.

57 NA: FD 1/1649. Fletcher to Griffiths, 23 May 1930.

58 NA: FD 1/1649. Fletcher to Dreyer, Hopkins, and MacNalty, 7 May 1930.

59 NA: MH 56/101. Robinson to Butcher, 15 December 1934.

60 Atkins, "White Heat in Whitehall."

61 *Parliamentary Debates,* 10 February 1931, cols. 891–8. This debate had been organized by Viscount Astor.

62 H.H. Scott, "Tuberculosis in Man and Lower Animals," *Medical Research Council, Special Report Series,* 149 (1930); John W.S. Blacklock, "Tuberculous Disease in Children," *Medical Research Council, Special Report Series,* 172 (1932); Lewis S. Jordan, "The Eradication of Bovine Tuberculosis," M*edical Research Council, Special Reports Series,* 184 (1933).

63 NA: MH 56/100; Sir Frederick Hopkins (chairman), *Report of the Economic Advisory Council on Milk Cattle Diseases*, British Parliamentary Papers 1933–34 (Cmd 4591), ix. 427.

64 Peter J. Atkins, "The Pasteurization of England: The Science, Culture and Health Implications of Milk Processing, 1900–1950," in David F. Smith and Jim Phillips (eds.), *Food, Science, Policy and Regulation in the Twentieth Century: International and Comparative Perspectives* (London: Routledge 2000), 37–51.

65 NA: FD 1/1649. Olga Nethersole died the following year.

66 Atkins, "Pasteurization of England"; Atkins, "'Your Enemy the Cow'"; Peter J. Atkins, "Getting into the In-tray: The Pre-history of a Policy Network: Pressure Groups and Bovine Tuberculosis, 1850–1950," unpublished ms., 2006b; Atkins, "White Heat in Whitehall"; Peter J. Atkins, "The Glasgow Case: Meat, Disease and Regulation, 1889–1924," *Agricultural History Review* 52 (2004): 161–82.

67 NA: CAB 58/185, Economic Advisory Council, Report, Proceedings and Memoranda of Committee on Cattle Diseases (EAC (CD) Series, 26–87), 1932–34, vol. 2, Memorandum no. 35: "Compulsory Pasteurization of Milk in Towns," stenographic notes of the evidence of the representatives of the Ministry of Agriculture and Fisheries, 14 December 1932.

68 NA: MAF/35/435. Dale to Blackshaw, 27 May 1933.

69 NA: MAF 35/554. Blackshaw, 21 September 1934.

70 NA: MH/56/85. Beckett to Maclachlan, 23 May 1935.

71 Ian Buchanan, *Michel de Certeau : Cultural Theorist* (London: Sage 2000), 89.

72 Bob Jessop, *State Theory: Putting the Capitalist State in Its Place* (Cambridge: Polity Press 1990).

73 Under the 1923 provisions, producers of Certified and Grade A (TT) milk had to have cows that were tuberculin-tested, with milk free from tuberculosis; the cows of Grade A and Grade A (Pasteurized) producers had to be inspected every three months by a vet and certified free of clinical tuberculosis.

74 Atkins, "Getting into the In-tray."

75 David Marsh and Martin J. Smith, "Understanding Policy Networks: Towards a Dialectical Approach," *Political Studies* 48 (2000):4–21.

76 Steve Hinchliffe, "Indeterminacy In-decisions: Science, Policy and Politics in the BSE Crisis," *Transactions of the Institute of British Geographers* 26 (2000):182–204, 194.

77 See Stanley Wasserman and Katherine Faust, *Social Network Analysis: Methods and Applications* (Cambridge: Cambridge University Press 1994); http://www.orgnet.com/sna.html (accessed September 2003); but for a critique see Mustafa Emirbayer and Jeff Goodwin, "Network Analysis, Culture, and the Problems of Agency," *American Journal of Sociology* 99 (1994): 1411–54.

10

At Home in the Colonies: The WHO-MRC Trials at the Madras Chemotherapy Centre in the 1950s and 1960s

HELEN VALIER

INTRODUCTION

Attitudes towards and treatment of communicable diseases changed considerably during the 1950s. New anti-malarials, the unprecedentedly powerful antibiotic penicillin, and the new anti- tuberculosis drugs were finally demonstrating the staggering – but as yet unfulfilled – potential of chemotherapy to challenge some of the world's most intransigent disease problems.[1] With the introduction of effective combined chemotherapy treatments, for instance using streptomycin, para-amino-salicylic acid (PAS), and isoniazid, came dreams of the total eradication of tuberculosis (a disease that though already in steep decline across the developed world was on the increase in many poorer countries). Chemotherapies promised treatments and cures for a range of illnesses that created terrible burdens of disability, physical and financial, for both individuals and societies.

The early dissemination of the first very effective anti-tuberculosis drug, streptomycin, has attracted the attention of historians for two reasons in particular: its initial phase of trialling and distribution was marked by considerable controversy, especially in Britain, where its scarcity and concerns over possible toxicity spawned tension and confusion between bureaucrats, the scientific and industrial communities, and the general public.[2] Moreover, it was the first drug subjected to "randomized controlled trial"; that is, the first drug for which a new statistical basis for participant selection was applied, replacing earlier systems of alternation between control and treatment groups.[3] Not every aspect of the introduction of streptomycin, however, has received the same degree of historical attention, nor have the other drugs with which streptomycin was combined (to so dramatically improve its curative potential) been much discussed. Yet the development of combined chemotherapy to treat tuberculosis in the developed world and its use as part of an emerging international collaborative effort to tackle the health crisis posed by tuberculosis in poor countries forms a crucial part of the global history of twentieth-century therapeutics and clinical research and as such deserves to be considered in depth.

Following the widespread introduction of streptomycin in the late 1940s (at a time of great optimism that the disease scourges of the world *would* be defeated by the agents of biomedicine), ongoing British tuberculosis chemotherapy research spawned an international research network of a size perhaps unprecedented in the history of medicine. It drew in several countries, notably in Britain's former colonies (and new Commonwealth partners) in India and Africa. Here, I examine two strands of this later phase in the life of streptomycin and anti-tuberculosis chemotherapy more generally. First, I consider how its use quickly became fraught with complications as doctors and medical scientists were faced with the new problem of rapidly developing bacterial resistance and the perennial problem of patient compliance with treatment regimes. Second, I explore how the international links founded between research and treatment centres in the developed and developing world generated a vibrant, if somewhat politically loaded, synergy.

Streptomycin was an exciting but very problematic drug for those involved in the treatment of tuberculosis. Its many toxic effects on the body were only part of the problem; of even greater concern was the production of streptomycin-resistant bacilli in a significant percentage of patients as a by-product of their treatment. Streptomycin-resistant strains of tuberculosis threatened not only to undo the good work of chemotherapy treatment in the individual but also to imperil the wider community in a new, potentially even more dangerous way. An urgent solution to the problem of resistance was required and was indeed vigorously pursued.[4] The introduction of combination chemotherapies making use of streptomycin in conjunction with PAS (discovered in 1946) or isoniazid (discovered in

1951) partly overcame problems of bacterial resistance and toxic reactions. As the drugs all worked in different ways, their simultaneous use in combination gave the bacillus much less time to mutate and grow resistant. The early use of these drugs was, however, far from straightforward. Combination therapies required extensive trialling to determine effective dosage, the extent of any toxic reactions, and the likelihood of complications arising owing to bacterial drug-resistance.

One obvious "market" for these new regimes of testing was the developing world, where tuberculosis was both more prevalent than in the developed world and on the increase. In the mid-1950s, a major testing facility was established in the Indian city of Madras,[5] combining the efforts of the British Medical Research Council (MRC), the World Health Organization (WHO), the government of Tamil Nadu, and the Indian Council for Medical Research (ICMR). This development has received little historical attention, with the notable exception of Sunil Amrith's recent account of the role of the Madras venture in early international health campaigns.[6] Amrith sets the concerns of the international development community somewhat against medical and clinical interests in tuberculosis. He characterizes the public health policies of WHO and others as driven by "cost-effectiveness" at the community level, whereas clinical interests tended to "individualize" the disease. Although Amrith's broad characterization is sound, a more detailed look at the clinical work and aspirations of the Madras facility reveals a great deal more about the priorities and needs of research biomedicine in the context of work in the developing world. Of crucial concern is how such overseas "laboratories" might effectively settle complex questions over the future use and effectiveness of the chemotherapeutic approach to disease eradication in the developed, as well as the developing, world.

The Madras centre was established with the aim of determining whether the use of chemotherapies could wholly negate the need for sanatorium care for sufferers from tuberculosis: in other words, to discover whether it was safe to treat tuberculosis in the domiciliary setting. At this time in the developed world, it was common for chemotherapy to be administered inside medical institutions alongside other treatments such as surgery, rest, therapeutic work, and so on, so trialling the drug for use as a mono-therapy and in the home was something quite new.

Further trials in Madras and in Nairobi, Kenya, tried to over-come the other main obstacle to tuberculosis eradication: lack of patient compliance and cooperation. Years of investigative effort were directed at discovering how short-course treatment using a variety of drug combinations and requiring minimal supervision could be implemented in both rich countries and poor countries. Such a treatment modality was expected finally to unleash the true potential of chemotherapy in the fight against tuberculosis.

In examining this reciprocal knowledge transfer between Britain and her former colonies, it is important to consider how the existing historical and anthropological scholarship addressing the colonial and postcolonial body and the discourses of colonial medicine might be used to contextualize the process of "exporting" research questions outside of the metropole in which they were conceived.[7] The Madras Centre, in keeping with MRC-WHO centres established elsewhere in the Commonwealth and in Eastern Europe, visibly addressed local needs and local concerns: domiciliary care clearly offered many benefits to Third World governments unable to afford to support systems of sanatoria. As Randall Packard has noted, such "top-down" eradication approaches championed by new post-World War II, post-colonial institutions like the WHO "brought about significant changes in the practice of colonial medicine ... [but] did not lay the groundwork for a relocalization of health systems, the reassertion of indigenous models, or even the development of a more effective integration of Western biomedical models with local knowledge and conditions ... [I]nternationalization of health moved the control and practice of health care even further from local settings."[8]

Moreover, the desire to seek answers to the intractable problem of tuberculosis in the developed world also informed the existence and activities of these research outposts. As such, they present a particularly fine example of the operation of colonial medicine during the decline of Empire and the incipiency of post-colonial relations.[9]

EARLY TRIALS OF TUBERCULOSIS CHEMOTHERAPY IN BRITAIN

The MRC's Tuberculosis Chemotherapy Trials Committee, formed in 1946, worked with a carefully selected group of physicians from across the country. All shared considerable experience in the assessment and treatment of tuberculosis patients and were keen to try out this new American therapy within the rigours of the newly defined and refined "clinical trial."[10] The choice to treat only patients with a very specific type of tuberculosis (defined as "acute progressive bilateral pulmonary tuberculosis of presumably recent origin, bacteriologically proved, unsuitable for collapse therapy, age group 15–25"),[11] patients unsuitable for forms of therapy other than bed rest, meant that random allocation to a control group treated with bed rest only was relatively unproblematic. The fact that tuberculosis was commonly monitored radiographically gave the committee and its researchers some means of independent objective assessment, since all x-ray films were submitted to the central committee along with case reports. All this meant that the committee's report in 1948, despite being based on only one hundred patients, was confident in its endorsement of streptomycin therapy as a great improvement on existing treatments, albeit only for one specific (not very common) kind of tuberculosis. The report urged immediate further research to determine the possible wider applicability of streptomycin and to investigate optimal dosage, ideal duration of treatment, and how to deal with drug-resistant bacilli.[12]

Following publication of the MRC's report and the subsequent wide dissemination of streptomycin, the British medical press cautiously welcomed the treatment as a therapeutic advance, though one beset by problems and risk.[13] As reported by the prominent chest physician Philip Ellman in the 1949 edition of the *Medical Annual* (a handbook for practitioners summarizing the year's developments), streptomycin therapy entailed many side-effects for patients, some very severe, and the emergence of streptomycin-resistant bacilli during treatment seemed unavoidable.[14] In addition, warnings issued by the MRC Trials Committee provoked widespread concerns that indiscriminate, inappropriate use might further exacerbate the likelihood of an explosive increase in drug-resistant forms of tubercle bacilli.[15]

In contrast to Ellman's description of the anxiety and uncertainty surrounding the publication of the first MRC streptomycin report is his depiction of the publication of the results of the MRC's trials of combined streptomycin and PAS therapy in 1950.[16] He extolled the latter as "[placing] the chemotherapy of this disease on a sound footing. Although many questions remain yet unanswered and the search for better drugs continues, a potent remedy is now at hand,

and much useful and proven information as to its effectiveness has emerged."[17] It was not just that PAS was itself a "potent" drug that pleased Ellman and others, however; rather, it was that its use revealed a means to overcome the knotty problem of bacterial resistance. While the MRC's study recognized PAS as a useable chemotherapeutic in its own right, it suggested that the real utility of the drug lay in the fact that when combined with streptomycin, many fewer cases of streptomycin-resistant tuberculosis arose as a result of chemotherapy treatment. Although PAS *could* be used alone, using it in combination brought about better results. Its use as a single agent was quickly restricted to streptomycin-resistant cases or to those showing toxic reactions to streptomycin.[18]

The effectiveness of combined chemotherapies in treating tuberculosis was considerably boosted through the widespread introduction of isoniazid in 1952. Although considerably more effective than either streptomycin or PAS, as a solo anti-tuberculous agent isoniazid, like streptomycin, had the unfortunate effect of producing drug-resistant bacilli in patients undergoing treatment. Once again a combined chemotherapy approach was deemed to be the answer. The effectiveness of the drug in combination (first with PAS or streptomycin and later with streptomycin and PAS) meant that a wider range of pulmonary tuberculosis and a growing number of chronic tuberculosis cases could now be treated with chemotherapy.[19]

Although chemotherapy use became more common during the early to mid–1950s, surgical, sanatoria, and bed rest treatments all remained prominent features of British approaches to tuberculosis.[20] The declining incidence of the disease led to the closure of many sanatorium beds, but the principles that underpinned sanatorium care – fresh air, rest, and good nutrition — remained firmly implanted in the mindset of clinicians dealing with tuberculous patients. Doctors in Britain were, therefore, reluctant to launch treatment trials using chemotherapy alone, especially for those cases in which the disease was much advanced. And when the Tuberculosis Society of Scotland launched a major study to question whether bed rest added value to chemotherapy treatment or whether it could be dispensed with, only "highly cooperative" patients with "mild forms" of the disease were chosen to participate in the study.[21]

For the most part, *ad hoc* clinical observation and personal impressions concerning the benefits of bed rest (or even a short period of sanatorium confinement) informed many of the discussions and trials of chemotherapies in Britain. Very little clear-cut data was produced on the benefits of single-modality therapeutic approaches, and, as in the Scottish trials, such data related only to specific forms of the disease. All this was dramatically changed by the MRC's work in Madras: operating under very different social and economic conditions, the team produced an avalanche of data that was at once conclusive and widely applicable. Aside from the (widely applauded) elegant design of the trial, such striking and clear-cut results were obtained in large part owing to the parlous state of India's health infrastructure, and more particularly its lack of sanatoria. The 1959 *Bulletin of the World Health Organization* noted that while India was estimated to have some one and a half million infectious cases of tuberculosis amongst its population, the numbers of sanatoria beds available for their care amounted to a mere twenty-three thousand.[22] This absence of viable alternative treatment regimes thus ensured that research programs in India and other poor countries were ostensibly less ethically problematic than those in the developed world.[23]

THE WHO, THE MRC, AND TUBERCULOSIS RESEARCH IN MADRAS, 1955–61

In 1955, at the request of the Indian government, the World Health Organization sponsored a visit to India by three MRC representatives: J.G. Scadding, P. D'Arcy Hart, and Wallace Fox. They were to advise on studies designed to provide information on the mass domiciliary application of chemotherapy in the treatment of pulmonary tuberculosis, as part of an ongoing plan to combat tuberculosis in the country.[24] Four years earlier, the WHO, in conjunction with the children's charity UNICEF and the government of India, had launched the National Tuberculosis Plan for India. The first phase of the plan (1951–56) was primarily concerned with providing the BCG vaccination to children. Efforts to impose an India-wide vaccination program continued into the second phase of the program (1956–61),[25] but to this effort was joined a new commitment to research (hence the invited presence of the MRC).[26] Following the visit, Fox and his co-workers were intimately involved in drawing up a WHO-Indian government plan for a tuberculosis research and treatment centre based in the city of Madras.[27] Teams under D'Arcy Hart and Ian Sutherland at the MRC's Tuberculosis Unit and Statistical Research Unit, respectively, planned out the initial trial protocol. While the Indian partners, especially the ICMR, were called upon to recruit local doctors, nurses, and other health workers, the overall design, execution, and analysis of the trial and trial data was managed by the MRC or by WHO-appointed men, such as Wallace Fox and Denis Mitchison, with strong ties to MRC units. Subsequent reports of the trials, however, put heavy emphasis on the importance of local expertise in ensuring patient compliance.[28] From monetary and food "inducements" for trial participants to family-wide education, unannounced home-urine checks, and ongoing cajoling, the persistence, ingenuity, and constantly evolving strategies of the Indian social workers, public health nurses, health visitors, and local doctors emerge as a crucial contribution to the overall success of the trial.

India's chronic lack of sanatorium beds made reliable domiciliary treatment an attractive alternative to the expense and disruption of sanatorium care. It was, however, an alternative accompanied by problems and risk. Sufferers participating in the study, drawn by the promise of free drugs and medical attention, might well drop out once they started to feel better. Individuals might develop, and then spread, drug-resistant strains of tuberculosis. And such an event, if common, could easily precipitate a massive public health crisis, overwhelming India's already struggling public health system. The design of the Madras tuberculosis trial took into account the difficulties of ensuring treatment compliance in the domiciliary setting. Mass domiciliary application was thus ruled out in the first instance. Rather, in creating a tuberculosis *centre* for the study in 1956, the collaborators sought to establish an investigator- controlled, centralized point of delivery and assessment.

The initial Madras research program comprised a twelve-month controlled comparative study of patients at home and patients in a sanatorium and follow-up of family contacts over a further four years. Patients were admitted to the program from an existing screening centre – the Government Tuberculosis Institute – in Chetput, at the heart of Madras (itself chosen as a representative large, very overcrowded city). In other words, participants were to be drawn from the pool of those attending a local centre after showing symptoms, that is, those in whom the disease was already quite advanced. It was considered important that patients should be selected in this way, as this was how the majority of cases in India presented. The centre took on a limited number of patients from elsewhere in the city, but nearly all came through the institute. These patients represented some of the city's poorest residents, living in some of the most overcrowded conditions.

The new Chemotherapy Centre was thus established adjacent to the existing institute in 1956, housed on a one-and-a-quarter hectare campus also owned by the government of Tamil Nadu.[29] In addition to building these new premises, the regional government also provided about forty staff members and one hundred sanatorium beds, and it agreed to meet 50 percent of the expenditure on a range of items. The Indian Council for Medical Research provided most of the rest of the money, as well as several medical, technical, and administrative staff members.[30] It was agreed that while the WHO would take overall control of the centre as part of the wider National Tuberculosis Plan, the MRC alone would be responsible for the planning and direction of scientific research at the facility.[31] Thus, although Fox was appointed as the head of the new Madras venture by the WHO, he was in reality a representative of the MRC, and he was the guiding figure in ensuring that the design and construction of the centre facilitated its use as a research facility.[32] The WHO also provided much of the initial apparatus and several key personnel to run the "routine" services in the Tuberculosis Demonstration and Training Section of the project.[33] The WHO and the Indian Government had originally agreed that all the centre's support services would be gradually taken over by the government of Tamil Nadu. The slow rate at which this transfer actually occurred, however, became a source of contention throughout the second phase of the National Plan.[34]

That the clinical locus of the trial was conveniently located next to the laboratory and administrative centres of the project greatly enhanced the likelihood of tight central control. There were two major requirements for patient selection to the Madras trial, both of which were assessed through strict interrogative interviews: the would-be patient should not have received previous chemotherapy (a fact that was in practice quite difficult to ascertain, since the free drugs attracted sufferers); and, furthermore, the individual had to be judged likely to comply with trial conditions (and ideally was able to show evidence of willingness from family members to be cooperative and supportive also). To become enrolled into the trial,

patients also had to be free of other chronic illnesses such as diabetes and leprosy and to be healthy enough to be considered for
home treatment. With such limited availability of sanatorium beds,
however, it seems very likely that consideration of quite what was
"healthy enough" for trial participation might have been significantly different in India than in the United Kingdom or other
developed countries.

In the trial itself, two series of patients – one group treated in sanatoria, one group treated at home – were given isoniazid and PAS
together. Clinically, the trial showed little percentage difference in
achieving bacteriological quiescence in home- versus sanatorium-
treated patients, though it did take the home group longer to begin
showing these results. In both the male groups under study, there
remained an intractable 10 percent of patients with active disease at
the end of twelve months, some of who also showed isoniazid-resistant tubercle bacilli in their sputum. Amongst the female study
groups, the sanatorium patients faired slightly better, although pre-
treatment discrepancies in general states of health were assumed to
have been the likely cause of this. The Madras study thus showed
that the results of combined isoniazid and PAS therapy could be as
effective in patients treated at home under very unfavourable conditions as it was in patients prescribed the identical chemotherapy in
the optimum environment of the sanatorium.

For the MRC, a professional self-interest in devising universally
applicable regimes of chemotherapy only (that is, regimes without
bed rest or sanatorium confinement), and multi-drug (or combined)
chemotherapy treatments was a strong motivating factor driving
tuberculosis research in India. Nonetheless, the Madras trials were
also designed to develop ways for poor countries to cope with their
own pubic health problems. In this, they can be considered successful: the trials clearly demonstrated the potential for low-cost treatments suitable for mass application. So should the Madras trials be
considered an exploitation of vulnerable clinical material or a practical and realistic attempt to disentangle the perennially intertwined
conditions of disease and poverty in poor countries?

One way to examine this balance of interests is to look at how the
ambitions and plans of the MRC compared with those of the WHO,
the government of Tamil Nadu, and the Indian Council of Medical
Research. A 1957 letter sent to the MRC-selected director of the
centre, Wallace Fox, from the WHO's head of the Communicable

Disease Division, Johs Holm, is revealing of possible conflicts between these competing interests:

> I understand your [Fox's] objectives for the project to be something like this: To study whether or not it is possible – when we have unlimited resources and facilities at our disposal, and if the patient may be given all types of refined examinations and receive any treatment that is available in the world today – to obtain as good results from treatment of patients in India as those experienced in the United Kingdom. You wish to do everything possible for each one of your patients, including those who have deteriorated after the treatment in the trial, to which they have been allocated; that is those patients who, for the purposes of the trial, can be described as failures and thereafter can be of little or no scientific interest. I realize that this is from humanitarian or, if you prefer it, clinical considerations and feelings.
>
> The objectives of the project as I see them – and I think the WHO in general – are somewhat different. They are to study the effect, in terms of rendering infectious patients non-infectious and keeping them so, of treatment that is inexpensive and which consists of self-administration of drugs with no close clinical supervision by experts and with no complicated laboratory tests ... I fully realize that in a scientific trial you sometimes have to use complicated methods and examinations (for example reliable resistance tests) but frankly I do not understand some of the arrangements you are making in your project, and I am afraid – as I have already told you personally – that by making the trial too complicated the purpose of the study will be defeated.[35]

Holm's comments show up an interesting distinction between MRC and WHO views on the importance of the trial at the individual level and at the community level. The concern of the WHO, as represented by Holm, was not so much with the individual infected with tuberculosis but, rather, with the prevention of spread of the disease. From the WHO's public health perspective, neutralizing the vectors of transmission, rather than curing sufferers, was the goal. Thus, the sometimes highly elaborate MRC preparations and persistent interest in curative therapies greatly frustrated the WHO.

The MRC researchers, for their part, often felt overly constrained by the WHO, especially with the organization's reluctance to allow their attendance at conferences and other scientific gatherings before full publication of results.[36] MRC relations with the ICMR also seem to have been less than smooth. In 1958, an emollient Fox wrote to his MRC colleague, Hart, to say: "It is my view that the MRC has failed to exploit the value of good personal relations or demonstrated that it has a 'human touch.' The Indian, in particular, responds to friendly gestures and doesn't like formal relationships à la British Raj."[37]

What the government of Tamil Nadu and the Indian Council of Medical Research thought of the project is less clear. The MRC files plainly state that friction between regional government and the WHO in India was nothing new, and as far as Fox was concerned, the issue to be addressed was how best the MRC could ease these traditional tensions.[38] As the centre matured, the Indian government began to insist that to have any long-term future it had to be staffed at the senior level by Indian nationals. Despite dire warnings from the MRC about the likely poor pool of candidates that would present itself following such a shift in policy, an "Indian takeover" of the project did indeed begin in 1964 with the appointment of N.K. Menon as centre director. The process was completed by the departure two years later of the last senior WHO figure, Hugh Stott.

CHEMOTHERAPY RESEARCH AND THE RECIPROCAL RELATIONS BETWEEN THE DEVELOPED AND THE DEVELOPING WORLD

Madras was the death knell for an increasingly moribund system of sanatorium treatment. But more than this, Madras showed definitively that the efficacy of chemotherapy was neither dependent on nor enhanced by a mixture of approaches. This caused a major shift in the clinical perception of tuberculosis. Writing his summary of recent developments in the treatment of pulmonary tuberculosis for the 1961 edition of *The Medical Annual*, J.R. Bignall reported in the most glowing terms on the implications of the Madras trials for rich and poor countries alike, musing, "It seems that it is not only rest that is unnecessary, but also *all that which for more than fifty years has been held to be essential in the mystique of treating tuberculosis.*"[39]

While Madras had shown convincingly that chemotherapy could overcome an adverse patient environment, a new, derivative series of studies aimed to use chemotherapy to negate an even larger problem concerned with the individual patient: the problem of compliance with therapy. During the initial Indian trial, it had been observed that a daily single dose of isoniazid could be used as an alternative to multiple, divided doses with little loss of efficacy and much potential for gain in terms of compliance and the ease and costs of administration. How to reap the benefits of this observation, while avoiding the complications that would follow the rise in the numbers of cases showing isoniazid-resistant bacilli, became a hot research topic. The Madras team (and later another MRC-linked team in Nairobi, Kenya) devised experiments to test whether, after a short period of daily supervised chemotherapy, an *intermittent* regimen of high-dose isoniazid, either given together with streptomycin or delivered alone, twice-weekly, under supervision and over a period of twelve months could be as effective and as safe as conventional therapy combination regimes.[40] Hart, in particular, was excited by this research because it was applicable to technically advanced counties including Britain, especially in overcoming problems of patient compliance and long-term cooperation.[41]

It is difficult to over-state the importance of compliance to the success of chemotherapies. Patients who took their medications erratically posed a risk not only to themselves but also, by becoming vectors for highly contagious antibiotic-resistant strains of the disease, to whole communities. Time and again, tightly controlled *trials* would achieve great successes, but when these protocols were transferred into the community and routine practice, their excellent results were not repeated.[42] A technical fix to the problem of compliance was, therefore, highly desirable in both developing and technically advanced countries.

Although their results were beneficial to the richer nations, a 1958 report to the MRC by the Madras Centre bacteriologist, D.A. Mitchison, made it quite explicit that the single-dose isoniazid Madras trial would never have been possible in the United Kingdom or in the United States, where standard treatment protocols were already in place:

The overseas schemes of the Council have provided most interesting problems and opportunities. Thus the studies in East

Africa and Madras on patients receiving isoniazid alone in different dosages could never have been carried out in Europe or America. They are likely to provide unique evidence on the significance of isoniazid resistance which remains a problem of the greatest importance in the field.

At least in the bacteriological field, it is clear that the overseas developments have been very successful and that they should be continued and even expanded. Whatever views are held on the importance of tuberculosis in Britain, the disease outside Europe and America remains one of the major scourges and will continue to present research problems for many years.[43]

The issues Mitchison raised are problematic and complex. It is clear that there was a wish to expand the MRC's overseas commitments in order to continue the MRC's ability to conduct research into tuberculosis. Similarly, the fact that trials that might be considered too risky or unethical in Britain were designed and run by British scientists in poorer, less-developed countries should also be examined with a critical eye. Nonetheless, the ethics of such activities must be considered in the context of British tuberculosis treatment of the time: many doctors did not want to change the dosage or duration of chemotherapy treatment. The Madras trials might have persuaded doctors that the sanatorium was no longer a necessary part of treatment, but their influence was not sufficient to eliminate prescriptions of bed rest followed by very long closely supervised courses of therapy, through which doctors could be certain that the tubercle bacilli had been destroyed.[44] Such attitudes militated against new home-based trials. Moreover, the policy of long duration follow-up observation in all cases swallowed resources and slowed efforts to redirect Britain's chest-clinics towards targeted management of "high-risk" groups.[45] Thus, the export of research overseas had perhaps more to do with evading the conservatism amongst clinicians at home and overcoming problems of "physician-compliance" than with trying out "dangerous" drugs and drug combinations on "subalterns."[46]

In 1950s Britain, tuberculosis remained common in the slums of the inner cities, stubbornly resisting the interventions of modern medicine. In such surroundings, poor general health and poor compliance with treatment regimes made tuberculosis a direct threat to the poor and thus a persistent, lurking threat to the whole nation.

As has been frequently observed by historians of empire, colonial indigenes were often likened to the working classes of the metropolitan cities.[47] Seen in this light, India's unhealthy poor were indeed excellent clinical material. It is worthy of note that the same 1959 edition of the World Health Organization's *Bulletin* that published results of the Madras trials also published a study directed at showing the potential to eradicate tuberculosis in the developed world using chemotherapy and close supervision: it targeted "high-risk groups" within poorer communities in Denmark.[48]

The usefulness of experimental results to Britain and similar countries should, of course, also be balanced against the benefits of this research to the populations and governments of host countries. For India, with virtually no sanatoria beds, the option to import MRC-trialled chemotherapies held the promise of a better, healthier future for huge numbers of ordinary people. On the other hand, the arrival of chemotherapies also reduced the urgency of solving the social and economic problems that underpinned this disease – poverty, overcrowding, and poor nutrition.

The MRC scientists in charge of these projects were well aware of the potential sources of complaint and criticism of their research overseas. Reflecting on his experiences in Madras and on the subsequent efforts to bring the Indian research findings to bear on the British context, Fox wrote in 1962:

I wish to describe how studies of tuberculosis undertaken in developing countries, with the specific object of investigating their problems, may also be valuable to countries with highly developed medical services, such as Great Britain. Because these studies are often undertaken in particularly challenging circumstances, such as unusually severe disease in a malnourished population, the findings may have especially wide applications. If a chemotherapeutic combination proves effective under very unfavourable conditions in a developing country, it is likely to be at least as effective in countries where the disease is, on average, less advanced, and the environmental factors are more favourable. In contrast, studies in medically advanced countries may be much less certain to be applicable in the developing world.[49]

Fox is candid about the fact that the background of desperate poverty made the chemotherapy research carried out at Madras

both clear-cut and generally applicable in a way that studies conducted elsewhere under better conditions simply would not have
been. Yet Fox is also adamant that such trials do no disservice to
the countries that host them or to the populations who participate
in them:

> Research in developing countries is not simply a question of
> applying information gained in the medically advanced commu-
> nities, such as Great Britain. Often it requires investigations in
> their own right of local problems. Equally research in develop-
> ing countries should not be regarded and approached as an
> opportunity to exploit areas with an abundance of clinical
> "material" in order to solve the problems of the medically
> advanced countries. Nonetheless, studies which break new
> ground scientifically may be of value not only to the developing
> countries for which they were undertaken but also for the tech-
> nologically advanced communities. Thus, a valuable reciprocal
> relationship can be established in which more-favoured and less-
> favoured countries helped one another.[50]

This principle of reciprocity underscored the work of Fox's
Madras Centre, as it would for the next phase of MRC trials examining intermittency and short-course combination chemotherapy
done in Madras and centres in East Africa and Hong Kong.
Although the imbalance of power between nations may have limited a true reciprocity, the huge effort on the part of the MRC to produce significant and enduring local change in overseas locations
and to employ rhetoric designed to show awareness of "colonial"
sensibilities is real enough. As such, it offers an intriguing insight
into nascent post-colonial relations within the Commonwealth in
the period immediately preceding the large-scale arrival of the pharmaceutical industry and marketplace in the developing world.

CONCLUSIONS: MADRAS AND A NEW BEGINNING FOR BRITISH COLLABORATIVE TUBERCULOSIS RESEARCH

The first Madras study was the beginning and cornerstone of a considerable upswing in British interest and institutional support for
tuberculosis research during a relatively quiet period for domestic

research in the United Kingdom.[51] The design of the centre itself showed the mechanisms by which strictly controlled trials meeting the highest of scientific standards could be conducted even in communities living under very poor circumstances. Following the successes of Madras, MRC involvement in tuberculosis research in Nairobi and Hong Kong flourished, as it did in several sites across Eastern Europe. Even with the so-called Indian take-over at Madras during the 1960s – the centre became the third permanent unit of the Indian Council of Medical Research in 1964 – MRC interests in India remained strong. This interest would decline only when subsequent appointments of Indian nationals to the staff created an environment in which ongoing MRC intervention in the running of the centre became less and less tolerated.

The significance of the Madras trials in terms of post-colonial relations is difficult to overstate. Here we have a continuation of the extractive and even exploitative model of colonial experimentalism, overlaid with an internationalist humanitarian development project. As the developed nations today cast worried eyes over domestic populations with ever-increasing levels of chronic illnesses such as type-II diabetes, HIV/AIDS, and indeed drug-resistant forms of tuberculosis, once again former colonies provide both abundant clinical material and an altogether different set of priorities that enable medical research to be conducted – and it should be said *ethically* conducted – according to an alternative set of rules.

NOTES

I would like to thank the Wellcome Trust for their support in this work, which was undertaken at the Wellcome Unit at the University of Manchester.

1 The trail of "disappointments" in the search for effective chemotherapy treatment of tuberculosis pre-streptomycin is told in Philip D'Arcy Hart, "Chemotherapy of Tuberculosis: Research during the Past 100 Years," *British Medical Journal* 2 (1946):805–10, 849–55. Similarly, the treatment of malaria between the wars can be characterized as a series of attempts to tackle the disease through synthesized drugs of relatively low efficacy when compared to existing natural remedies. For a discussion of chemotherapy treatment of malaria see George M. Findlay, "Malaria: Modern Treatment," *Medical Annual: A Yearbook of Treatment and Practitioner's Index* (1949): 201–8, 201.

2 For discussion of the introduction of streptomycin and surrounding controversies see Alan Yoshioka, "Streptomycin in Postwar Britain: A Cultural History of a Miracle Drug," *Clio Medica* 66 (2002): 203–27; and Milton Wainwright, "Streptomycin: Discovery and Resultant Controversy," *History and Philosophy of the Life Sciences* 13 (1991): 97–124.

3 Lise Wilkinson, "Sir Austin Bradford Hill: Medical Statistics and the Quantitative Approach to Disease," *Addiction* 92 (1997):657–66; and Alan Yoshioka, "Use of Randomisation in the Medical Research Council's Clinical Trial of Streptomycin in Pulmonary Tuberculosis in the 1940s," *British Medical Journal* 317 (1998):1220–3. Yoshioka questions the extent to which the trial should be considered as truly novel in this regard and considers the wider social and political context of centrally controlled randomization.

4 Medical Research Council, "Streptomycin Treatment of Pulmonary Tuberculosis," *British Medical Journal* 2 (1948):769–82, discusses the problem of streptomycin-resistant bacilli arising in patients treated with the drug (and for this reason urges caution in the use of streptomycin) and calls for immediate investigations directed at overcoming this obstacle to treatment (see especially 781).

5 Madras was officially renamed Chennai by the Indian government in 1996.

6 Sunil Amrith, "In Search of a 'Magic Bullet' for Tuberculosis: South India and Beyond, 1955–1965," *Social History of Medicine* 17 (2004):113–30. See also idem., *Decolonizing International Health: India and Southeast Asia, 1930–65* (New York: Palgrave Macmillian, 2006).

7 See, for instance, David Arnold, *Colonizing the Body: State Medicine and Epidemic Disease in Nineteenth Century India* (Berkeley: University of California Press 1993); Andrew Cunningham and Bridie Andrews (eds.), *Western Medicine as Contested Knowledge* (Manchester: Manchester University Press 1997); Mark Harrison, *Climates and Constitutions: Health, Race, Environment and British Imperialism in India, 1600–1850* (Oxford: Oxford University Press 1999).

8 Randall Packard, "Postcolonial Medicine," in John Pickstone and Roger Cooter (eds.), *Medicine in the Twentieth Century* (London: Harwood Academic Publishers, 2000), 97–112, 100.

9 David Jones, "The Health Care Experiments at Many Farms: The Navajo, Tuberculosis, and the Limits of Modern Medicine, 1952–1962," *Bulletin of the History of Medicine* 76 (2002): 749–90, examines similar relations in the American context in which "Researchers exploited the opportunities made possible by the ill-health of a marginalized popula-

tion, but did so with the cooperation and gratitude of the Navajo" (749) during the 1950s.

10 Medical Research Council, "Streptomycin Treatment," 769–70. There were various toxicity scares surrounding streptomycin, and a good deal of hype and anti-hype accompanied its testing phase (for details see Yoshioka, "Streptomycin in Postwar Britain"). Nonetheless, the trial itself recruited well and progressed smoothly.

11 Medical Research Council, "Streptomycin Treatment," 770.

12 Ibid., 780–1.

13 As described in the summary reports of the current literature carried by the *British Medical Annual: A Yearbook of Treatment and Practitioner's Index* for the period.

14 Philip Ellman, "Tuberculosis, Pulmonary: Treatment," *Medical Annual: A Yearbook of Treatment and Practitioner's Index* (1949):368–73, 371.

15 Ibid., 371.

16 "Treatment of Pulmonary Tuberculosis with Streptomycin and Para-Aminosalicylic Acid: A Medical Research Council Investigation," *British Medical Journal* 2 (1950):1073–85.

17 Ellman, "Tuberculosis, Pulmonary: Treatment," 319.

18 Ibid., 320.

19 "Treatment of Pulmonary Tuberculosis with Isoniazid: An Interim Report to the Medical Research Council by Their Tuberculosis Chemotherapy Trials Committee," *British Medical Journal* 2 (1952):735–46.

20 J.L. Livingstone, "On the Treatment of Tuberculosis at the Present Time," *British Medical Journal* 1 (1955):243–50.

21 D.T. Kay, "The Treatment of Pulmonary Tuberculosis at Work: A Controlled Trial. An Interim Report by the Research Committee of the Tuberculosis Society of Scotland," *Tubercle* 38 (1957):375–81; and Report from the Research Committee of the Tuberculosis Society of Scotland, "The Treatment of Pulmonary Tuberculosis at Work: A Controlled Trial," 41 (1960):161–70. As will become clear later, the fact that this second publication followed but made no mention of the MRC studies in Madras was a cause for derision, not least from the MRC. See Philip D'Arcy Hart, "Treatment with Rest," *Tubercle* 41 (1960):397.

22 Tuberculosis Chemotherapy Centre, Madras, "A Concurrent Comparison of Home and Sanatorium Treatment of Pulmonary Tuberculosis in South India," *Bulletin of the World Health Organization* 21 (1959):51–131, 51. The cited source for this figure is ICMR, Special Report Series 34 (1959), 75.

23 Jones's discussion of the Navajo trials of isoniazid during the early 1950s shows that many of these concerns and considerations were mirrored in

the U.S. context and that clear-cut clinical material – i.e., individuals previously untreated with antibiotics suffering from a specific type of tuberculosis (in the case of these experiments cases of miliary tuberculosis were sought) – was becoming a scarce commodity as more of the general population was exposed to chemotherapy ("Tuberculosis Research and the Navajo," 763.) The cases are also analogous in that the Navajo reservations were able to provide few sanatorium beds, and little public health infrastructure to their impoverished residents.

24 Tuberculosis Chemotherapy Centre, Madras, "Comparison of Home and Sanatorium," 52.

25 These "phases" are described in "The National Tuberculosis Plan, India. June 1959," UK Public Records Office (PRO), FD 7/1020.

26 It seems likely that MRC staff were themselves very active in stimulating interest in an India-based tuberculosis research program involving the council. Denis Mitchison, a prominent co-worker of Wallace Fox, recently described how he and Fox would negotiate the establishment of such programs with public health figures in WHO and foreign governments. (Comments made at the Wellcome Trust, History of Twentieth Century Medicine Group, "Short Course Chemotherapy for Tuberculosis," Witness Seminar, London, 3 February 2004.)

27 Drafts of this plan annotated by MRC staff can be found in the PRO, FD 7/1020 files.

28 Tuberculosis Research Centre, Madras, "History of the Tuberculosis Research Centre," http://www.trc-chennai.org/history/htm (accessed 13 March 2002).

29 Ibid.

30 "WHO/Indian Government Tuberculosis Trial, 14/11/55–22/9/59, agreement between the World Health Organisation and the Government of India," PRO, FD 7/1020.

31 Ibid.

32 Philip D'Arcy Hart to Arthur Landsborough Thomson, 26 April 1956, PRO, FD 7/1020, describes the council's nomination of Fox to head the project.

33 Details in FD 7/1020 files.

34 Details in FD 7/1020 and FD 7/1021 files.

35 Johs Holm to Wallace Fox, 25 April 1957, PRO, FD 7/1022. This source is also cited and quoted in the article by Amrith, in which he draws a similar conclusion within a different context. See Amrith, "In Search of a 'Magic Bullet.'" 124.

36 In a letter from the MRC's P. D'Arcy Hart to Harold Himsworth in London, Hart claimed that because of the restrictions placed on him by the WHO, Fox was able to get to the annual International Tuberculosis Conference only by what amounted to "a subterfuge" (22 September 1959, PRO, FD 7/1022). Such complaints are repeated elsewhere in the files.

37 Wallace Fox to Philip D'Arcy Hart, 27 December 1958, PRO, FD 7/1020.

38 Ibid.

39 John R. Bignall, "Tuberculosis: Rest and Pulmonary Tuberculosis," *The Medical Annual* (1961): 429–31, 430, my emphasis.

40 For some early MRC work on combination chemotherapy in East Africa, see East African/British Medical Research Council, "Comparative Trial of Isoniazid in Combination with Thiacetazone or a Substituted Diphenylthiourea (SU 1906) or PAS in the Treatment of Acute Infectious Pulmonary Tuberculosis in East Africans," *Tubercle* 41 (1960):399–423.

41 Philip D'Arcy Hart to Harold Himsworth, 17 May 1963, PRO, FD 23/1088.

42 Editorial, "Shorter Chemotherapy in Tuberculosis," *Lancet* 299 (1972):1105–6, 1005. This issue was discussed at length at the Wellcome Trust Witness Seminar, "Short Course Chemotherapy for Tuberculosis."

43 Denis Mitchison, "Summary of Work of Present Groups, c.1958," PRO, FD 371/62968.

44 A 1961 report by the British Tuberculosis Association recommended long-term supervision, possibly life-long supervision, of all patients treated with chemotherapy for their tuberculosis. See "Relapse in Pulmonary Tuberculosis: An Analysis of the Fate of Patients Notified in 1947, 1951 and 1954: Report from the Association's Research Committee," *Tubercle* 42 (1961): 178–86. For comments on the drawbacks of long-term supervision see East African/British Medical Research Councils, "Controlled Clinical Trial of Short-Course (6-Month) Regimens of Chemotherapy for Tuberculosis: First Report," *Lancet* 299 (1972):1079–85; "Third Report," *Lancet* 304 (1974):237–40.

45 In a letter to the *Lancet* Fox and Mitchison described non-cooperative groups as commonly comprised of "alcoholics, vagrants and migrants," (308 [1976]:1349–50, 1349). Other "high-risk" groups of patients might be those suffering a serious co-morbidity (such as diabetes) or those living with the after-effects of major surgery. See S.J. Pearce and N.W. Horne, "Follow-Up of Patients with Pulmonary Tuberculosis Adequately Treated by Chemotherapy: Is It Really Necessary?" *Lancet* 304 (1974):641–3, 642.

46 This is not to say that the toxicity of certain drugs and the possible reck-lessness of chemotherapy trials in nurturing drug-resistant strains were not issues of concern for those participating in or observing the research. They were. What I suggest here is that the export of clinical trials was not by necessity underpinned by any "sinister" motive but was rather an effort to break down clinical attitudes that had become widely entrenched.

47 See Mark Harrison, Climates and Constitutions, and David Arnold, Colonizing the Body.

48 E. Groth-Petersen, Jorgan Knudsen, and Erik Wilbek, "Epidemiological Basis of Tuberculosis Eradication in an Advanced Country," Bulletin of the World Health Organization 21 (1959):5–49.

49 Wallace Fox, "The Chemotherapy and Epidemiology of Tuberculosis: Some Findings of General Applicability from the Tuberculosis Chemo-therapy Centre, Madras," Lancet 280 (1962): 413–17, 473–8, 413.

50 Ibid., 477.

51 For a discussion of the rapid decline in interest in tuberculosis amongst the British medical population by the early 1960s, see Anne Hardy, "Reframing Disease: Changing Perceptions of Tuberculosis in England and Wales, 1938–1970," Historical Research 76 (2003): 535–56, 554; and Linda Bryder, Below the Magic Mountain: A Social History of Tuberculosis in Twentieth Century Britain (Oxford: Clarendon Press 1988), 262–3. As Hardy notes, "Even the emergent concern over tuberculosis amongst Asian immigrants did not regenerate enthusiasm for the problems of the disease." ("Reframing Disease," 555).

Contributors

Peter J. Atkins, University of Durham, England

David S. Barnes, University of Pennsylvania, United States

Alison Bashford, University of Sydney, Australia

Tim Boon, Science Museum, London, England

Linda Bryder, University of Auckland, New Zealand

Flurin Condrau, University of Manchester, England

Jorge Molero-Mesa, Universitat Autònoma de Barcelona, Spain

Helen Valier, University of Houston, United States

John Welshman, Lancaster University, England

Michael Worboys, University of Manchester, England

Index

venereal diseases, 172
ventilation, 150
vibromassage, 30
Virgin Mary, 30
virgin soil, 125, 137–42, 158–62

wage structure, 178
waiting list, 78
Waksman, Selman, 4, 75
Wartime Social Survey, 41
water supply, 150
Weber, Max, 92, 149
Weighall, Archibald, 200
welfare reform, 172
Wellingborough, 124
Welsh National Medical School, 159
West Bromwich, 132
Weybridge, 197

WHO, 7, 113, 117, 213–34
Williams, Robert Stenhouse, 191, 200
Williams, Tom, 202
Wilson, Graham Selby, 191, 200
Wolverhampton, 132, 139
Wood, H. Kingsley, 199
work therapy, 30, 76, 81
working conditions, 161, 171
working-class biographies, 82, 86
Wright, Norman, 200

x-rays, 10, 39, 41, 107–11, 115–16, 126–36, 141–2, 217

yaws, 130
yellow fever, 130

zoonosis, 205